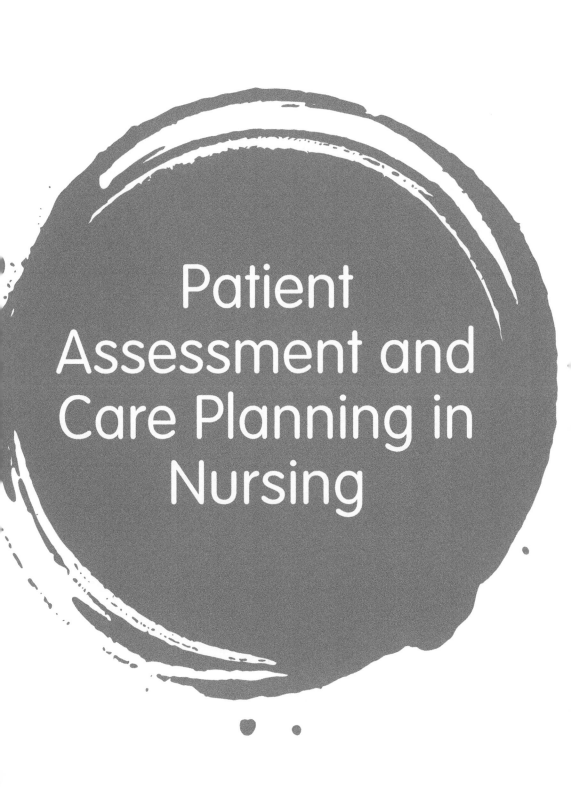

Patient Assessment and Care Planning in Nursing

Sara Miller McCune founded SAGE Publishing in 1965 to support the dissemination of usable knowledge and educate a global community. SAGE publishes more than 1000 journals and over 800 new books each year, spanning a wide range of subject areas. Our growing selection of library products includes archives, data, case studies and video. SAGE remains majority owned by our founder and after her lifetime will become owned by a charitable trust that secures the company's continued independence.

Los Angeles | London | New Delhi | Singapore | Washington DC | Melbourne

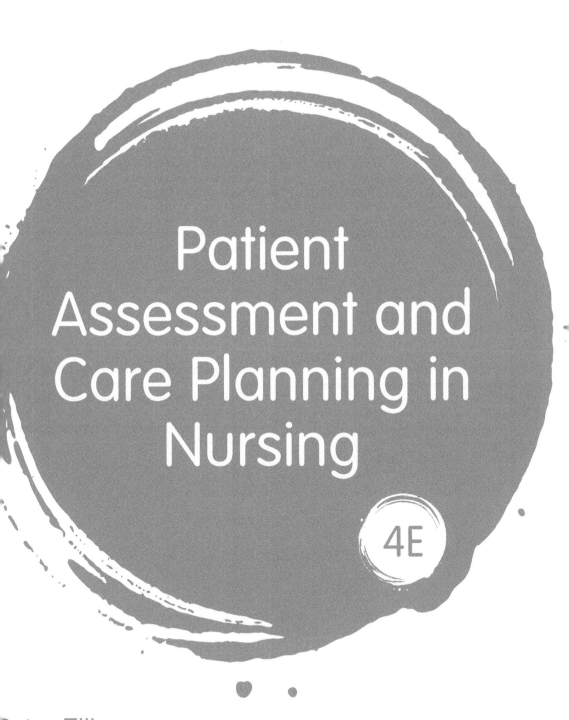

Patient Assessment and Care Planning in Nursing

4E

Peter Ellis

Mooi Standing

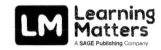

Learning
Matters
A **SAGE** Publishing Company

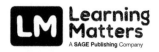

Learning Matters
A SAGE Publishing Company
1 Oliver's Yard
55 City Road
London EC1Y 1SP

SAGE Publications Inc.
2455 Teller Road
Thousand Oaks, California 91320

SAGE Publications India Pvt Ltd
B 1/I 1 Mohan Cooperative Industrial Area
Mathura Road
New Delhi 110 044

SAGE Publications Asia-Pacific Pte Ltd
3 Church Street
#10-04 Samsung Hub
Singapore 049483

Editor: Martha Cunneen
Development editor: Richenda Milton-Daws
Senior project editor: Chris Marke
Project management: River Editorial
Marketing manager: Ruslana Khatagova
Cover design: Sheila Tong
Typeset by: C&M Digitals (P) Ltd, Chennai, India

Library of Congress Control Number: 2022948441

British Library Cataloguing in Publication data

A catalogue record for this book is available from the British Library

ISBN 978-1-5296-0999-8
ISBN 978-1-5296-1000-0 (pbk)

Contents

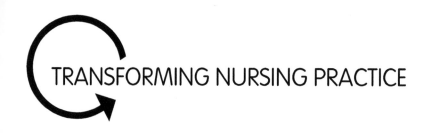

TRANSFORMING NURSING PRACTICE

Transforming Nursing Practice is a series tailor made for pre-registration student nurses. Each book in the series is:

- Affordable
- Mapped to the NMC Standards of proficiency for registered nurses
- Full of active learning features
- Focused on applying theory to practice

Each book addresses a core topic and has been carefully developed to be simple to use, quick to read and written in clear language.

An invaluable series of books that explicitly relates to the NMC standards. Each book covers a different topic that students need to explore in order to develop into a qualified nurse... I would recommend this series to all Pre-Registered nursing students whatever their field or year of study.

LINDA ROBSON,
Senior Lecturer at Edge Hill University

Many titles in the series are on our recommended reading list and for good reason - the content is up to date and easy to read. These are the books that actually get used beyond training and into your nursing career.

EMMA LYDON,
Adult Student Nursing

ABOUT THE SERIES EDITORS

DR MOOI STANDING is an Independent Nursing Consultant (UK and International) and is responsible for the core knowledge, adult nursing and personal and professional learning skills titles. She is an experienced NMC Quality Assurance Reviewer of educational programmes and a Professional Regulator Panellist on the NMC Practice Committee. Mooi is also Board member of Special Olympics Malaysia, enabling people with intellectual disabilities to participate in sports and athletics nationally and internationally.

DR SANDRA WALKER is a Clinical Academic in Mental Health working between Southern Health Trust and the University of Southampton and responsible for the mental health nursing titles. She is a Qualified Mental Health Nurse with a wide range of clinical experience spanning more than 25 years.

BESTSELLING TEXTBOOKS

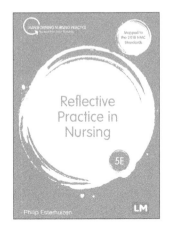

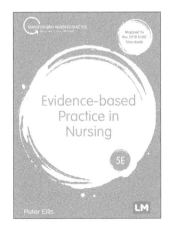

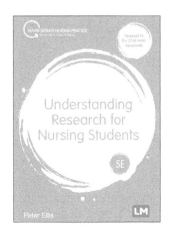

Reflective Practice in Nursing

Evidence-based Practice in Nursing

Understanding Research for Nursing Students

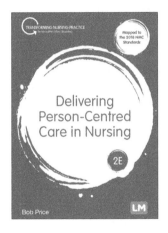

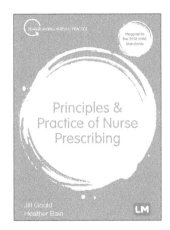

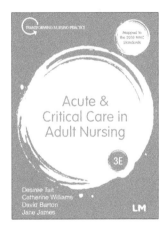

Delivering Person-Centred Care in Nursing

Principles & Practice of Nurse Prescribing

Acute & Critical Care in Adult Nursing

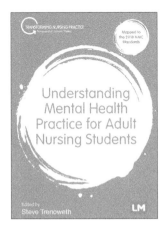

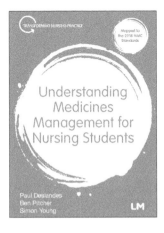

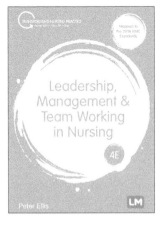

Understanding Mental Health Practice for Adult Nursing Students

Understanding Medicines Management for Nursing Students

Leadership, Management & Team Working in Nursing

You can find a full list of textbooks in the *Transforming Nursing Practice* series at
https://uk.sagepub.com/TNP-series

About the authors

Peter Ellis is an independent nursing and health and social care writer and consultant, and CEO of Intelligent Care Software. Peter was most recently a Registered Manager and Nursing Director in the hospice and social care settings. Prior to this, he was a senior lecturer and programme director at Canterbury Christ Church University where he taught patient assessment and care planning, among other topics, to undergraduate and postgraduate students. Peter is also an Honorary Senior Research Fellow of Canterbury Christ Church University and has a special interest in palliative and end-of-life care.

Dr Mooi Standing is an Independent Nursing Consultant (UK and International) and is responsible for the core knowledge, adult nursing and personal and professional learning skills titles. She is an experienced NMC Quality Assurance Reviewer of educational programmes and a Professional Regulator Panellist on the NMC Practice Committee. Mooi is also a Board member of Special Olympics Malaysia, enabling people with intellectual disabilities to participate in sports and athletics nationally and internationally.

Acknowledgements

To all of our patients, clients and residents who are the inspiration for this book. Our gratitude and thanks to Lioba Howatson-Jones, who was the primary author of the early editions of this book and to Sue Roberts who authored a chapter on community health needs assessments in previous editions. We would also like to thank all our readers who have taken the time to provide us with their invaluable feedback to date, which has helped us in enhancing this current edition.

Introduction

Who is this book for?

The new, updated edition of this book is for all student nurses, and other health and social care professionals, who wish to develop their assessment and care planning practice and for novice practitioners who wish to extend their understanding of practice. This edition of the book has seen the removal of the chapter which specifically focused on patient assessment, preventative healthcare and health promotion in the community setting. Instead, these themes are now incorporated throughout the book, with examples from across a wide variety of health and social care settings, demonstrating the process and practice of patient assessment and care planning in nursing.

What is patient assessment?

Patient assessment is a process that identifies and defines the problems which patients (and other service users) present with, in order for solutions to be planned and implemented in line with their preferences. The purpose of this book is to introduce student nurses and other health and social care practitioners to the different stages of the assessment and care planning process. It also raises some of the considerations which need to be thought about within decision-making, such as the inclusion of the service user and an emphasis on person-centredness. The book takes a holistic approach to patient assessment, which means that it looks at what is happening with the patient as part of a whole, including socially, mentally and spiritually, rather than concentrating on purely physical aspects of patient assessment and care planning.

The role of the nurse in assessment continues to evolve as nurses take on new roles within health and social care. In order to prepare for the future you need to be ready to recognise both the commonality and the complexity of assessment across different settings and within changing health and social care provisions. The health and social care agenda is shifting to involve people more in the assessment, planning and delivery of their own care. In each of the chapters you will be given opportunities for integrating your learning through the worked examples and scenarios, which include assessments of people of all ages experiencing a variety of mental and physical problems. You will also be encouraged to examine the involvement of other health and social care practitioners.

The structure of the book

Chapter 1 sets all that follows firmly within the context of person-centred care. This chapter introduces us to the 6Cs of nursing and identifies your values and beliefs in relation to person-centred assessment and practice, before giving you some practical pointers for building upon these beliefs and putting them into action.

Chapter 2 explores the understanding of our role in patient assessment. It considers the factors that promote or inhibit effective patient assessment and looks at how to build on your current skills and knowledge of what patient assessment means. You will be asked to examine how attitudes, beliefs and stereotyping can affect the accuracy of patient assessment, and how to balance subjective and more objective forms of assessment.

Chapter 3 explores some of the different techniques needed for making sense of patient information. The chapter defines what patient information is and identifies the roles of different health and social care professionals in gathering patient information. You will be encouraged to try out different questioning techniques and to differentiate between different types and forms of information and how to analyse these in order to identify nursing priorities.

Chapter 4 examines the purpose of assessment tools and looks at a range of assessment tools including the Malnutrition Universal Screening Tool (MUST), Waterlow, and the National Early Warning Score 2 (NEWS 2). You will be asked to reflect on the knowledge and skills needed to use assessment and screening tools and consider some potential problems of focusing purely on the tool. You will explore how to use information gained from screening and assessment to achieve a nursing diagnosis and a plan of care.

Chapter 5 defines what is meant by nursing diagnosis. It includes the history and development of nursing diagnosis and explores how it relates to the patient assessment process. You will be asked to examine the potential benefits and problems of nursing diagnoses for the patient and health and social care professionals. You will also be encouraged to practice developing a nursing diagnosis from a patient assessment.

Chapter 6 examines why care plans are necessary and how to identify a nursing problem. You will be asked to examine the care planning stages and identify short- and long-term goals and determine interventions. You will consider examples of different care plans and be given an opportunity to develop a written care plan of your own.

Chapter 7 introduces the relevance of nursing models to the care planning process. In this chapter we will examine why models are important and look at a variety of nursing models. You will be encouraged to think about how a nursing model frames the patient assessment process and how the nursing model impacts on decision-making in care planning. In this chapter, you will see how nursing models can work together with the nursing process to enable nurses to generate some sample care plans.

Chapter 8 introduces some of the ethical aspects of patient assessment. You will be asked to develop your understanding and application of ethics within patient assessment processes by reviewing ethical principles such as autonomy, beneficence, non-maleficence and justice. You will be encouraged to examine the relevance of ethical theories to patient assessment by considering some ethical challenges in patient assessment and resource allocation. This is followed by an exploration of some problems with ethics in theory and ethics in practice.

Chapter 9 examines how patient assessment informs clinical judgement and decision-making. It relates patient assessment to Standing's (2023) ten perceptions of clinical decision-making in nursing (collaborative, observation, systematic, standardised, prioritising, experience and intuition, reflective, ethical sensitivity, accountability, and confidence), cognitive continuum theory (nine modes of practice), and 'PERSON' evaluation tool. It explores how the issues discussed in Chapters 2–8 can be addressed by applying the ten perceptions of decision-making and nine modes of practice to patient assessment and decisions about patient care. The 'PERSON' evaluation tool emphasises the importance of continually reassessing and evaluating nursing decisions to ensure that they are patient-centred, promote safe and effective care, and identify areas for improvement.

The glossary at the end of the book explains specialist terms in plain English.

Requirements from the NMC Standards

Evidence-based nursing requires the nurse to have knowledge and skills, which are outlined in detail in the document *Future Nurse: Standards of Proficiency for Registered Nurses* (Nursing and Midwifery Council, NMC, 2018a). These standards are used by educational institutions when planning professional courses. They are grouped into seven 'Platforms', as shown in the box below.

NMC Future Nurse: Standards of Proficiency for Registered Nurses

Platform 1: Being an accountable professional

Registered nurses act in the best interests of people, putting them first and providing nursing care that is person-centred, safe and compassionate. They act professionally at all times

(Continued)

(Continued)

and use their knowledge and experience to make evidence-based decisions about care. They communicate care effectively, are role models for others, and are accountable for their actions. Registered nurses continually reflect on their practice and keep abreast of new and emerging developments in nursing, health and care.

Platform 2: Promoting health and preventing ill health

Registered nurses play a key role in improving and maintaining the mental, physical and behavioural health and well-being of people, families, communities and populations. They support and enable people at all stages of life and in all care settings to make informed choices about how to manage health challenges in order to maximise their quality of life and improve health outcomes. They are actively involved in the prevention of and protection against disease and ill health and engage in public health, community development and global health agendas, and in the reduction of health inequalities.

Platform 3: Assessing needs and planning care

Registered nurses prioritise the needs of people when assessing and reviewing their mental, physical, cognitive, behavioural, social and spiritual needs. They use information obtained during assessments to identify the priorities and requirements for person-centred and evidence-based nursing interventions and support. They work in partnership with people to develop person-centred care plans that take into account their circumstances, characteristics and preferences.

Platform 4: Providing and evaluating care

Registered nurses take the lead in providing evidence-based, compassionate and safe nursing interventions. They ensure that the care they provide and delegate is person-centred and of a consistently high standard. They support people of all ages in a range of care settings. They work in partnership with people, families and carers to evaluate whether care is effective and the goals of care have been met in line with their wishes, preferences and desired outcomes.

Platform 5: Leading and managing nursing care and working in teams

Registered nurses provide leadership by acting as role models for best practice in the delivery of nursing care. They are responsible for managing nursing care and are accountable for the appropriate delegation and supervision of care provided by others in the team, including lay carers. They play an active and equal role in the interdisciplinary team, collaborating and communicating effectively with a range of colleagues.

Platform 6: Improving safety and quality of care

Registered nurses make a key contribution to the continuous monitoring and quality improvement of care and treatment in order to enhance health outcomes and people's experience of nursing and related care. They assess risks to safety or experience and take appropriate action to manage those, putting the best interests, needs and preferences of people first.

Platform 7: Coordinating care

Registered nurses play a leadership role in coordinating and managing the complex nursing and integrated care needs of people at any stage of their lives, across a range of organisations and settings. They contribute to processes of organisational change through an awareness of local and national policies.

This book draws from these standards and presents the relevant ones at the beginning of each chapter.

Activities

At various stages within each chapter there are points at which you can break to undertake activities. Undertaking and understanding the activities is an important element of your comprehension of the content of each chapter. You are encouraged, where appropriate, to reflect on your practice and consider how the things you have learned from working with patients, and others, might inform your understanding of patient assessment and care planning. Other activities will require you to take time away from the book to find out new information which will add to your understanding of the topic under discussion. Some activities challenge you to apply your learning to a question or scenario to help you reflect on issues and practice in more depth. A few activities require you to make observations during your day-to-day life or in the clinical setting. In some cases, you are encouraged to discuss your thoughts or findings with a mentor or one or more fellow students. All the activities in this book are designed to increase your understanding of the topics under discussion and how they impact upon nursing practice.

Where appropriate there are suggested or potential answers to activities at the end of the chapter. It is recommended that you try, where possible, to engage with the activities in order to increase your understanding of the realities of patient assessment and care planning.

Chapter 1

Person-centred assessment and practice

Peter Ellis

NMC Future Nurse: Standards of Proficiency for Registered Nurses

This chapter will address the following platforms and proficiencies:

Platform 1: Being an accountable professional

At the point of registration, the registered nurse will be able to:

1.9   understand the need to base all decisions regarding care and interventions on people's needs and preferences, recognising and addressing any personal and external factors that may unduly influence their decisions.

Platform 3: Assessing needs and planning care

At the point of registration, the registered nurse will be able to:

3.4   understand and apply a person-centred approach to nursing care, demonstrating shared assessment, planning, decision making and goal setting when working with people, their families, communities and populations of all ages.

3.5   demonstrate the ability to accurately process all information gathered during the assessment process to identify needs for individualised nursing care and develop person-centred evidence-based plans for nursing interventions with agreed goals.

Chapter aims

After reading this chapter, you will be able to:

- identify your values and beliefs in relation to person-centred assessment and practice;
- assess how you might work in ways that are person-centred;
- discuss the 6Cs and how they relate to person-centred practice;
- identify what is meant by person-centred workplace cultures; and
- develop strategies to introduce person-centred and 6Cs-based practice.

Case study: Ella's experience of someone living with learning disability

Ella was a second-year midwifery student completing a placement in a high-risk birthing centre. Her supervisor, Breed, was a highly experienced midwife. Ella still had a number of objectives to achieve in order to progress to the third year, including empowering diverse service users, and she discussed this with Breed as part of her learning contract discussion. A phone call interrupted their discussion and Breed took details. When Breed had finished the conversation, she informed Ella that a woman called Mandy was coming by ambulance with a difficult birth presentation, and that she had a learning disability.

Ella was concerned about how she would communicate with Mandy as she had no experience of dealing with people with learning disabilities. She imagined that Mandy would be terrified, with no idea about what was happening to her. Ella also imagined that Mandy would probably have difficulty processing detailed information.

Mandy arrived with her mother, Ruby, who was looking distressed. Ella immediately went to reassure Ruby that they would help Mandy as quickly as possible while Breed got ready to examine Mandy. Breed ascertained that Mandy's baby was a shoulder presentation requiring a caesarean delivery and contacted the obstetrician and anaesthetist immediately. Throughout this, Mandy was crying in pain and Ella tried to help calm her, but Mandy was getting cross. Ella tried to explain what they were doing but realised that she was using medical terms that Mandy did not understand. She felt helpless but persevered by asking Mandy to tell her what she was experiencing. The obstetrician arrived, completed her assessment and explained the process for proceeding to caesarean to Ruby and asked her to sign the consent. Ella observed how Ruby explained to Mandy what was happening before going with her to theatre. Mandy's baby was a large baby boy, who she named Liam.

Afterwards, when taking a break in the coffee room, Ella listened to the midwives discussing Mandy's case. A number wondered how Mandy would cope with a baby. One midwife, Miranda, said that it was not fair on the baby. Others argued that Mandy had the support of her mother and that some women were not as fortunate as that. Ella found herself thinking that Mandy would need a lot of support because of her learning disability.

Introduction

Working in person-centred ways is fundamental to the provision of good quality care. Its absence is often identified in health and social care organisations that are failing. As is highlighted in the case study, however, some staff working in health and social care hold values and beliefs that are not person-centred and are likely to influence both the way they practise and the quality of care within the organisations in which they work. This chapter will begin by providing some background to the quality improvement agenda in the UK and then proceed to identify some definitions of what person-centredness is, and why it is so important. The chapter will outline the importance of developing awareness of our own values and beliefs and how these contribute to the ways in which we work both as individual nurses and to the wider workplace culture. The chapter will conclude with some strategies to help you develop person-centred ways of working that also encompass the now-famous 6Cs.

Background to quality improvement in health and social care in the UK

Deficits in care and compassion have been identified in a number of high-profile reports about failures to provide the requisite level of care to patients or service users in a number of health and social care organisations (Equality and Human Rights Commission, 2011; Francis, 2013; Keogh, 2013; Care Quality Commission (CQC), 2022). These issues are not confined to England but appear in the rest of the UK as well, although they are often explained as isolated incidents (Andrews and Butler, 2014) despite statistics for healthcare complaints rising sharply (Northern Ireland Public Services Ombudsman, 2021; Scottish Public Services Ombudsman, 2022). For context, in 2020/2021, the NHS in England received 170,013 complaints (NHS Digital, 2022), or 300 per 100,000 of the population; and this despite a pause to the complaints process between March and June 2020 due to COVID-19.

Indeed, healthcare failures are a worldwide problem (WHO, 2018). Notably, many of the failures and complaints relate not to care per se, but more often to the ways in which care is delivered, poor communication and lack of information giving (NHS Digital, 2022).

Such figures about failures in care and the attendant complaints do raise the question: what is going on with care that makes it so bad? This question could also be more specifically directed towards nursing, which is singled out as a problem in many of the care failure reports. The most influential response came from the Chief Nurse for England, Jane Cummins, who, with the Department of Health, in 2012, developed a vision of compassion in practice for nursing, midwifery and care staff. This was rolled out to all NHS staff from 2014 by NHS England (Stephenson, 2014). This vision sets out the core values needed to underpin practice, which are commonly known as the 6Cs. They are:

Care

Care is nursing's core business and that of our organisations; the care we deliver helps both the individual patient or client and improves the health of the whole community. Caring defines us and our work. People receiving care expect it to be right for them, consistently, throughout every stage of their life.

Compassion

Compassion is a measure of how care is given through relationships based on empathy, respect and dignity. It can also be described as intelligent kindness and is central to how people perceive their care. When compassion is lacking, it interferes with the relationship between nurses and patients and can give rise to complaints.

Competence

Competence means all those in caring roles must have the ability to understand an individual's health and social care needs. They must also have the expertise, clinical and technical knowledge to deliver effective evidence-based care and treatments.

Communication

Communication is central to successful caring relationships and to effective team working. Without communication, there can be no person-centred care. Listening to what patients and clients want is essential to support notions such as 'no decision about me without me' (Department of Health, 2010a). Communication is the key to a person-centred workplace culture that benefits both those in our care and staff.

Courage

Courage enables us to do the right thing for the people we care for, to speak up when we have concerns (Rahman and Myers, 2019), and to have the personal strength and vision to innovate and to embrace new ways of working, perhaps even when other staff are resisting.

Commitment

A commitment to our patients and populations is a cornerstone of what we do. We need to build on our commitment to improve the care and experience of our patients and take action to make this vision and strategy a reality for all and meet the health, care and support challenges ahead.

What this means in practice is treating the people we care for in a kindly way, with dignity and respect, listening to their wishes and advocating for them when required (NMC, 2018a). This requires confidence in ourselves, in our profession and in each other to do the right thing. Blaming a lack of time or resources is not an acceptable reason for poor practice. Throughout the chapters in this book, you will be asked to review some of the case studies to identify which of the 6Cs are most applicable to the case. In this way, you will be able to become familiar with interpreting how the 6Cs play out in practice.

While a lack of resources and leadership coupled with a rising workload are very real issues for health and social care organisations, there appears to be a fundamental shift within some individuals who are employed by them, which apparently leads to uncaring attitudes and behaviours. While some of this may, over a period of time, be put down to compassion fatigue – where the ability to cope becomes overwhelmed (Sorenson et al., 2016) – some research suggests that the barriers to care are not the nurses and carers themselves, but the failure of organisations and society to adapt to an increasing social care model in the healthcare setting (Baumbusch et al., 2016). The Francis Report specifically calls for improvement in care and compassion as well as greater emphasis on involving people in decisions about care (Francis, 2013). Similarly, Scotland is focusing its healthcare improvement work on collaborating with people, their families and carers, bringing people together through, for example, the People-Led Care Portfolio (Health Improvement Scotland, HIS, 2021), which focuses on understanding people's experiences of care in their own words gathered by having meaningful conversations with people. Similar ventures are developing in Northern Ireland and Wales. However, it is encouraging that lessons appear to have been learned from the seismic Francis Report, through a change in emphasis from competency to the inclusion of caring attitudes and behaviours in quality audits. You are encouraged to complete Activity 1.1 to consider a different perspective.

Activity 1.1   Reflection

Watch the following video clip: **www.youtube.com/watch?v=XOCda6OiYpg**

How would you want to respond to the quality concerns raised previously?

There are some outline suggestions at the end of the chapter.

Within your answer to the activity, you might have considered your professional values and what your profession does well, and how you want to portray this to others. You might see some parallels in the narrative within the poem and how people responded to the selfless work of nurses, and other key workers, during the COVID-19 pandemic.

We move on now to consider what person-centredness is.

What is person-centredness?

In order to define person-centredness, we need to first consider: what is a person? Some define personhood as grounded in feelings of *being in the world* (Heron, 1992), while others suggest that such a being has rational capability and basic moral status or human rights (Ikäheimo and Laitinen, 2007), or more broadly possesses attributes that make them a person (Dewing, 2008). Carl Rogers, a well-known psychologist and humanist, argues that person-centredness is a way of being that sees the whole person embedded in their lifeworld (Rogers, 1995). What this means is that we need to recognise that people do not just exist but are fashioned and created as a result of important, and some seemingly less important, events and interests in their lives as well as by the people around them and how they relate to the world as a whole. Such interests are both physical (e.g. being fed and warm) and psychosocial and spiritual (e.g. being treated with respect and dignity and being recognised as an autonomous being) (Ellis, 2020). Who we are and how we see the world, the person we are, is therefore tied up in our experiences and relationships. Building therapeutic relationships with people uses values of respect, empathy, empowerment and being genuine. You might like to complete Activity 1.2 to consider what makes you the person you are.

Activity 1.2   Reflection

Consider the following:

- Who are the people you are connected with?
- What are the significant events in your life?
- What is important to you?

Based on your answers above, what kind of person do you consider yourself to be? Have there been events in your life which have changed who you are when perhaps you least expected them to?

As this activity is based on your personal experience, there is no outline answer at the end of the chapter.

Consequently, if our ideas about what a person is are connected to how we interact with 'persons' in the world, what does being person-centred mean? Person-centredness has long been debated in the literature and has often been used interchangeably with similar terms such as patient-centredness, which confuses the issue. Some definitions of person-centredness and person-centred care can be found in Table 1.1.

What these definitions have in common is respect, trust and a support for the right to self-determination. This can be enabled by practice development activities, which explore ways of working differently and critically help you reflect on how you are involved in your practice and with patients (or, should we say, people?). Often the starting point is an analysis of the language you use to describe your practice and patients/service users. This can reflect your values and beliefs about person-centredness, which is what we move on to consider now.

Person-centredness	*A standing or status that is bestowed upon one human by others, in the context of relationship and social being. It implies recognition, respect and trust.*
	(Kitwood, 1997, page 8)
	Person-centredness is an approach to practice established through the formation and fostering of healthful relationships between all care providers, … people [service users] and others significant to them in their lives. It is underpinned by values of respect for persons, individual right to self-determination, mutual respect and understanding. It is enabled by cultures of empowerment that foster continuous approaches to practice development.
	(McCormack et al., 2013, page 193)
Person-centred care	*Care that: is focused on clients/users; promotes independence and autonomy rather than control; involves services that are reliable and flexible and chosen by users; and tends to be offered by those working in a collaborative/team philosophy.*
	(Innes et al., 2006, page ix)
	An approach to practice established through the formation and fostering of healthful relationships between all care providers, service users and others significant to them in their lives. It is underpinned by values of respect for persons, individual right to self-determination, mutual respect and understanding. It is enabled by cultures of empowerment.
	(McCormack and McCance, 2016, page 20)
	Person-centred care moves away from professionals deciding what is best for a patient or service user, and places the person at the centre, as an expert of their own experience. The person, and their family where appropriate, becomes an equal partner in the planning of their care and support, ensuring it meets their needs, goals, and outcomes.
	(Social Care Institute for Excellence, ND)

Table 1.1   Definitions of person-centredness and person-centred care

A good example of the use of language in this respect is the change from referring to people as 'asthmatics' or 'dementia patients' to 'people living with asthma' and 'people living with dementia'. What this language identifies is a focus on the person first and the disease second – person-centred language.

Identifying values and beliefs

You will have developed your own values and beliefs through reflection on your upbringing, life experiences and the people you interact with. Identifying your own values and beliefs is an important starting point for self-awareness and, as we described earlier, for personhood. To identify your own values and beliefs, you first need to be clear what a value is and what a belief is. Some consider values to represent the authentic self in terms of identity behaviours (Stets and Carter, 2011), while others suggest that values can shift over time (Morris, 2012). One of the leading commentators on values, Schwartz (1992), describes values as being the beliefs that are attached to a desirable outcome of a particular action; values themselves are more important than any given situations, and therefore give us the ability to choose between different ways of behaving and the outcomes associated with them. Schwartz further suggests that people rank values according to what is important to them, and as such these values motivate our behaviours both as individuals and within societies.

Beliefs, on the other hand, are our convictions about the way we see things regardless of what the evidence is telling us. Kahneman (2011, page 209) makes the observation:

> *For some of our most important beliefs, we have no evidence at all, except that people we love and trust hold these beliefs. Considering how little we know, the confidence we have in our beliefs is preposterous—and it is also essential.*

Notably then, there is no necessary logic to our values and beliefs and as a result, and as Morris (2012) suggests, they can change over time. It is down to us as nurses however to choose the influences we allow to shape what we value and believe.

Through making explicit our values and beliefs, we are taking the first steps to making them a reality in the ways in which we practise and within the cultures of the workplace. Congruence between what we say we believe and how we act is one of the hallmarks of effective individuals, teams and organisations (Manley, 2000) and is one of the reasons that student nurses often go through a sea-change in how they see the world and what they value and believe during their training as they try to make sense of new experiences.

Activity 1.3   Critical thinking

You are now invited to complete a values clarification exercise to explore your values and beliefs about person-centredness. This may take you approximately 30 minutes. A values clarification exercise is a grand title for a simple exercise designed to access and clarify the values and beliefs we hold about something. For the purpose of developing an understanding of person-centredness, you are being asked to consider the following statements:

- I believe the ultimate purpose of person-centredness is …
- I believe this purpose can be achieved by …
- I believe the factors that inhibit or enable this purpose to be achieved include …
- Other values/beliefs that I hold about person-centredness are …

You might like to list three or four fundamental values that underpin your beliefs and guide your actions and behaviours. Once you have completed the exercise, make a note of any questions you are asking yourself. This exercise is adapted from Manley and McCormack (2003).

As this activity is based on your personal ideas, there is no outline answer at the end of the chapter.

It is important to understand our own values and beliefs because when we meet people who are different from us, we can temper the ways in which we act by recourse to our own values and beliefs, rather than being influenced by the behaviours of others, which may not be desirable. Similarly, we can identify people who share our values and beliefs and learn from the ways in which they behave and act, as you might do with your practice educator. This in turn may lead you to adopt new values, or adapt your existing values, so that they reflect the values of nursing as identified in the 6Cs.

That all said, there is no one right set of values and beliefs, rather, there are many values and beliefs which are to be regarded as worthy of respect and, conversely, many which are not. Recognising and valuing someone else's perspective, their values and beliefs, is a key aspect of being person-centred and of starting to understand different cultures and ways of being, including those of the workplace.

Workplace culture

Culture is experienced as a social phenomenon involving people in different ways. Manley et al. (2011, page 4) state that workplace culture is:

> *The most immediate culture experienced and/or perceived by staff, patients, users and other key stakeholders. This is the culture that impacts directly on the delivery of care. It both influences and is influenced by the organisation and corporate cultures with which it interfaces as well as other idiocultures through staff relationships and movement.*

Idiocultures are the behaviours and knowledge that a group of people hold and with which they interact. A group that works together may have settled into a particular way of thinking and behaving, which they do unconsciously, and into which they **acculturate** new members. For example, the case study at the start of this chapter hints at a kind of midwifery workplace culture that might exist. Some of these hints (such as the assumptions made about how Mandy, who lives with a learning disability, might cope) appear in the discussion in the coffee room. You are invited to think more deeply about workplace cultures and what culture means to you in Activity 1.4.

Activity 1.4   Critical thinking

Begin this activity by thinking about what words might be used to describe a workplace culture. You might consider using ideas such as describing the culture of the place you most recently worked as an animal, a colour, or perhaps a car, describing why you have chosen to describe the culture in the way that you have. When generating your answer, consider how you might explain it to a room of people.

When you have described your workplace culture, enter the word 'culture' into Google and consider the results. How do these compare and contrast to your ideas?

Now think about how culture is formed and who has the greatest influence on its development, and what you think (from your experience) makes it good or bad. List the attributes of both.

There is an outline answer at the end of the chapter.

You might have thought about a workplace where you felt everyone worked really well together or one where there was tension and disagreement. The important thing is to be able to critically analyse the elements of each so that you can recognise what the attributes are. Consider the following case study and answer the questions at the end to help develop your thinking.

Case study: Rob's observation of workplace culture

Rob was a radiography student completing a sampling placement on a care of the older person ward. He was only there for a week. His collaborative practice module in university had covered some theory relating to workplace culture, and for his assignment he needed to observe a workplace culture that was different from his own. Rob thought that this sampling placement would provide him with a good opportunity to observe the workplace culture in this area. He discussed this with the ward manager, Martin, who was keen to hear about his observations as he was trying to make some changes.

On his first day, Rob was welcomed by Julie, an older nurse who was approaching retirement. She spoke about this often. She said she loved the job but that it was getting harder with all the changes and new technology. After showing Rob round, Julie introduced him to other members of the team. She also introduced him to some of the patients she seemed particularly fond of. However, Rob noted the contrast when a member of staff from another ward came to ask about borrowing something. Julie was quite sharp in her response. The same happened when one of the kitchen staff came to say that a patient had spilled water on the floor.

Rob observed that the ward smelt fresh and was reasonably tidy. The clinical room seemed almost regimented in its order. He was assigned to accompany a healthcare assistant called Judith while she completed patient vital sign observations. He noted that she wheeled the observation machine from patient to patient and that she called them all 'duck' while explaining what she was doing. Other staff did not appear concerned about this and the patients appeared to respond positively.

During a coffee break, Rob listened to the conversation in the staffroom. It was mostly about what people were planning to do at the weekend or on future holidays. However, one part of dialogue caught his attention when Julie started to talk about the changes Martin was making to the ward. Although Julie could see the need for progress, she felt that 'old-timers'

(Continued)

15

(Continued)

such as herself were not consulted, despite their years of experience. Julie looked around the staffroom for support, and May, a nurse who usually worked nights, started to snipe about Martin. Rob decided to leave the room at this point.

At lunchtime, Rob observed Martin leading the shift handover. There was some chat at the start about unrelated issues and then the relevant nurses handed over their patients. Rob noticed that the language used was very medically oriented, with little comment on how people might be feeling. The handover was predominantly about the tasks that had been fulfilled.

Rob made a few notes about his observations to help with his assignment preparation. What was of greater concern to him at present was how he was going to feed back his observations to Martin, as he did not want to appear to have been 'spying'.

1. What observations do you think Rob is likely to have made about this ward culture?
2. In what way is Rob feeling uncomfortable about providing Martin with feedback?
3. How might Rob present his feedback?

There are some outline answers at the end of the chapter.

What the case study shows is that workplace culture is something which can cause you to respond in ways that are contrary to your **values** and beliefs as other factors come into play, such as power and authority. It also shows that workplace culture is dynamic and not fixed, and therefore can be changed by the participants – it is also notable that more than one culture was in evidence. Therefore, if you, as a participant in the workplace, are thinking and working in person-centred ways, you can make a positive contribution to your workplace culture by influencing how others think and behave.

Person-centred ways of working

Being person-centred in our working means first of all developing person-centred thinking in the way we communicate with others and how we frame our practice. This can be difficult when healthcare systems appear to be committed to standardising practice, reducing the opportunities for getting to know patients as people (McCormack et al., 2013). You need to be prepared to use the time you have to attentively listen to what people are saying – whether patients or staff members – and develop empowering ways of problem-solving that support positive ways of working. Attentive listening involves the following:

- a facilitative attitude that shows trust in the person's potential;
- attending, observing and listening, showing you're 'being with' someone – this might be called *sympathetic presence;*
- processing what you have heard by thoughtfully searching for meaning; and
- being aware of your internal dialogue, checking for potential actions or assumptive obstacles.

(Egan, 2014)

Doing this requires you to focus on finding solutions *with* people rather than dwelling on problems that maybe they can do nothing about. Being solution-focused means interpreting things differently, with an emphasis on positive elements, such as the strengths and resources that people bring from their lives to achieve their goals (Lynch et al., 2008). The person, not the problem, is at the centre of enquiry. The person's ideas, language and expertise are privileged, and their way of being *with* persons is proactive rather than reactive (McAllister, 2007). For this type of thinking, you need to use imagination and creativity as well as reasoning. Their motivation is likely to increase because you are building on people's strengths, rather than emphasising their weaknesses, as you generate personal plans. In this way, both the person and the health professional take responsibility to try creative solutions. Consider the following case study and then answer the questions at the end in order to help you develop some person-centred practice solutions.

Case study: Helen's hair solution

Helen is a mental health nurse working in a unit with older persons, many of whom are living with dementia. Last week, she admitted June. June had been living alone, with neighbours doing what they could to help her as she had no living family. However, when she arrived, she appeared very unkempt, with extremely knotted hair and stained clothing. Helen had gently settled June into the unit with a hot drink and gave her options for what she wanted to do. It was clear that June was disorientated.

This week, June has appeared more settled, until anyone tries to go near to brush her hair, when she starts to scream and becomes very agitated. Helen sits down with June and asks her whether she liked going to the hairdresser. June starts to talk about when she was a teenager with a beehive hairdo, getting admiring looks from the boys. Her hair was her pride and joy until there was a house fire at home and she was seriously injured. She remembered how horrible she looked with burned hair. It took months for her hair to grow back. She doesn't like people touching it!

Helen asked June if she had any photos of her beehive hair. June said she had a small one in her bag. Helen looked at it with June. She said she knew a lady called Maureen who was really good at doing hair and asked June if she wanted to meet her. June mumbled, 'Maybe'. Helen arranged for Maureen to come in at the end of the week and asked Maureen to first show June what she could do with Helen's hair. She noted a spark of interest from June when Maureen started working on Helen's hair. When Maureen had finished, Helen asked June if she wanted Maureen to help her with her hair and what she wanted doing. June responded positively, and Maureen was able to gently release the tangles from June's hair and create a lovely style for her. Helen and June compared their styles at the end and had a good laugh together.

(Continued)

(Continued)

1. How does Helen's care delivery compare or contrast with what we have discussed in this chapter?
2. How does what Helen did compare to what you would do?
3. How can you develop imaginative thinking about finding solutions with persons?

There is an outline answer at the end of this chapter.

Activity 1.5   Critical thinking

Look back at the 6Cs and then at the case studies in this chapter. Can you identify which of the 6Cs are actively evident in the case studies?

There is an outline answer at the end of the chapter.

Chapter summary

This chapter has explored the concepts of the 6Cs and person-centredness with regard to values, beliefs and workplace culture, and explored more positive ways of working with people that encourage motivation and collaboration. Through the activities, you have been given opportunities to identify your own values and beliefs and definitions of culture, in order to help you understand how you can adopt the 6Cs into and develop your person-centred practice further.

Activities: brief outline answers

Activity 1.1   Reflection (page 10)

You might have considered how members of your profession show how they care on a day-to-day basis, showing compassion and respect for patients/clients/service users, with some specific examples. You might also have thought about writing your own poem or narrative to show this.

Activity 1.4   Critical thinking (page 14)

You might have thought that culture meant a shared set of behaviours or seeing things in similar ways to others. Examples of a culture as an animal might be a 'lion culture', where the staff are fearless in the defence and support of the people they care for. Your culture might be a 'Ford Mondeo' (nothing special, but reliable and always gets the job done) or a colour such as blue (everyone is always upset or downhearted).

When Googling the word 'culture', you might have discovered diverse meanings, such as 'a group of people sharing certain characteristics and acting on certain assumptions'. People who have the most influence on the formation of cultures are often the leaders, who set the tone that others follow, or are perhaps the most vocal, who always influence the ways in which others think and behave.

Your list of attributes for good cultures might have included self-awareness, clarity of roles and priorities, insight into the consequences of actions, giving and receiving effective feedback, high challenge and high support, and teamwork and open communication. Your list of attributes for bad cultures might have identified working individually, lack of clarity of roles, unclear priorities, closed communication, little or no feedback, and high challenge with low support.

Case study: Rob's observation of workplace culture (page 15)

Rob is likely to have observed the inconsistent welcome given to different people, which reflects how they are viewed by members of the ward team. He is also likely to have observed the use of non-person-centred language to patients and staff and the task-based approach to care and talking about care. This reveals that regardless of what the ward philosophy might be, the care experienced by patients and staff is not person-centred. Rob is likely to feel uncomfortable because he feels some of the socialisation effects from the conversation in the staffroom, and he now has to show that he does not want to be socialised to think as the group do. On the other hand, he also does not want to be socialised into Martin's way of working either, being uncomfortable with the adoption of a medical- and task-oriented model of care. Rob is likely to feel uncomfortable because in providing feedback to Martin, he is likely to feel that he is not being authentic. Rob might present his feedback as the observations of an outsider. In this way, he might align himself to a more neutral patient role.

Case study: Helen's hair solution (page 17)

Helen's care is based on getting to know June as a person – being person-centred – through talking about areas of her life that she is able to remember. We don't know what the culture on the unit is, or what Helen's values are specifically, but the fact that she is willing to take time to get to know June suggests that the culture might be supportive to working in person-centred ways and that Helen's values are about respecting persons. You might be more used to task-based care plans that are mainly physically focused, or you may be very familiar with working out solutions with people. The way to develop imaginative thinking is to take a risk, as Helen did when asking June about her previous hairdresser experience. Through such gentle probing, solutions may start to emerge in creative ways.

Activity 1.5   Critical thinking (page 18)

The first case study involving Ella and Mandy demonstrates use of care and communication. The case study involving Rob shows commitment and courage. The case study involving Helen and June demonstrates commitment, compassion and courage to innovate.

Further reading

Francis, R (2013) *Report of the Mid Staffordshire NHS Foundation Trust Public Inquiry: Executive Summary*. Available at: www.midstaffspublicinquiry.com/sites/default/files/report/Executive%20summary.pdf

The official report into the failings at Mid Staffordshire Hospitals trust.

Keogh, B (2013) *Review into the Quality of Care and Treatment Provided by 14 Hospital Trusts in England: Overview Report*. Available at: www.nhs.uk/NHSEngland/bruce-keogh-review/Documents/outcomes/keogh-review-final-report.pdf

This report was ordered by the then prime minister following the findings of the Francis Report, and looked at 14 hospitals that had high death rates.

Kitwood, T (1997) *Dementia Reconsidered: The Person Comes First.* Milton Keynes: Open University Press.

Core reading about caring for people living with dementia.

Manley, K, Sanders, K, Cardiff, S and Webster, J (2011) Effective workplace culture: the attributes, enabling factors and consequences of a new concept. *International Practice Development Journal*, 1(2): Article 1.

The write-up of a long-term action research study into cultures in the workplace.

Price, B (2022) *Delivering Person-Centred Care in Nursing.* (2nd edn). London: SAGE.

A book which does what the title says and is well worth reading.

Rosen, M (2021) *Many Different Kinds of Love: A Story of Life, Death and the NHS.* London: Ebury Press.

The story of a survivor of COVID-19 and of the NHS staff who cared for him – person-centred care from the patient's viewpoint.

Useful websites

www.bacp.co.uk

Although this website is predominantly aimed at counsellors, it has some useful reading around the person-centred and solution-focused approaches (see types of therapy) and will also be helpful to those working in other fields, particularly mental health.

www.helensandersonassociates.co.uk

This website offers a variety of resources and examples of person-centred practice with different groups of people, including child, adult and mental health nurses.

www.cqc.org.uk/guidance-providers/regulations-enforcement/regulation-9-person-centred-care

One of the regulations guiding care from the Social Care Act 2008 (Regulated Activities) Regulations 2014 as inspected for by the Care Quality Commission.

Chapter 2

Understanding our role in patient assessment

Peter Ellis

Chapter aims

After reading this chapter, you will be able to:

- identify the nurse's role in patient assessment and discuss why it is so important;
- describe four ways of knowing and the nature of truth;
- use Standing's cognitive continuum and identify its relevance to nurses and patient assessment; and
- understand some consequences of stereotyping.

Introduction

Case study: Mr Tyler's dog bite

Mr Tyler keeps a number of very large dogs. One of them recently bit him on the left hand while he was trying to separate a dog fight in his back garden. Mr Tyler attended the local minor injuries unit, where he had the wound cleaned and dressed and was given a tetanus booster and a course of antibiotics.

You are on placement with the community district nurses, who have been asked to check the wound and continue the dressings as necessary. Mr Tyler answers the door and you are faced by a man who has numerous piercings and tattoos and who is wearing a death metal T-shirt. You feel quite intimidated. Before you can clean the wound, the old dressing has to be removed, and it appears quite dirty. The district nurse asks Mr Tyler what he has been doing to get the wound dressing so dirty. Mr Tyler starts to get angry. The district nurse tries to calm him by saying that until she knows what his needs are, she cannot offer any potential solutions to keep the wound clean. Mr Tyler identifies that he repairs motorbikes and needs to use both hands to do this, and he cannot take time off as he has a number of projects due for completion. The district nurse suggests that he could wear gloves while he does this and identifies where he might buy these. She also emphasises the importance of keeping the wound clean in order to help it heal. She explains that the healing process will take longer because Mr Tyler is still using his hand. Afterwards, you ask if she felt intimidated. The district nurse explains the importance of meeting people where they are. Her priority is assessing the individual's needs rather than imposing an ideal solution.

The case study above highlights the importance of courage – one of the 6Cs – as you confront your fear and focus on the person instead (to review the 6Cs, see Chapter 1). In the previous chapter, you were asked to explore your values and beliefs around person-centredness. Our values can also form part of the framework for patient assessment. The Nursing and Midwifery Council's code of professional standards of practice and behaviour for nurses, midwives and nursing associates (NMC, 2018b) clearly states the values nurses are expected to apply within their professional work. Nurses come from different cultural contexts and backgrounds where their own individual value systems will have started to develop. It is important to recognise the origins of your own attitudes and beliefs and how these will influence how you see things, especially how they might affect the way in which you undertake patient assessments.

The case study above highlights how someone's dress and personal presentation can be interpreted as reflecting values and beliefs that may be very different from yours, and you may find this challenging and potentially intimidating. How you feel can influence not only how you behave, but also the way you frame your patient assessment, and may also affect how much time it takes. It is important, as the case study identifies, to work with the patient in planning their care. What is most important here is that the assessment is about the patient's health needs, not about who they are or what they believe. This chapter will explore factors that may promote or inhibit effective patient assessment. It will also look at how to build on your current skills and knowledge (learnt both in nursing and outside) to develop your patient assessment technique. It will begin by clarifying what patient assessment means and then continue by considering how attitudes, beliefs and stereotyping can affect the accuracy of patient assessment, and how to balance subjective and objective forms of assessment.

What is patient assessment?

Properly done, patient assessment is the *holistic* process of evaluating the patient's mental, physical, social, cultural, spiritual and personal needs, and of identifying the patient's wishes in relation to the options available for meeting these needs. Failure to recognise and respond to patient needs can result in those needs not being met and a failure of care (McCormack and McCance, 2016; Wilson et al., 2018). This will be detrimental to the patient and may be professionally damaging for health professionals caring for the patient, including you. For example, you may not pass the practice assessment component of your programme. Within patient assessment, it is important to consider the patient's *lifeworld* in order to identify that patient's needs. Lifeworld refers to the history, culture, people, relationships and situations that are part of a patient's experience (West et al., 2007). The following case study helps to illustrate these points.

Case study: Graham's medical ward placement

Graham was in the second year of his nurse preparation programme, working on a ward specialising in diabetes care. Sam, a student undertaking a law degree, was newly diagnosed with diabetes and was struggling with managing his blood sugar level control. Graham was asked by his practice supervisor, Brett, to complete Sam's admission assessment.

Graham checked Sam's notes before meeting him and identified that he had had two hypoglycaemic episodes in the last few days, the most recent being one that brought him to accident and emergency.

Graham asked Sam about his medical history and then checked his understanding of diabetes. He noted that Sam was a vegan and that he had been given advice from the dietitian previously. Graham assumed that Sam would therefore know what foods he could have and those he needed to take care with. Sam told Graham that he had completed his exams recently, which he thought might have contributed to his hypoglycaemic episodes, due to the stress affecting his eating pattern.

(Continued)

(Continued)

Graham completed the assessment, documenting Sam's veganism in the biographical section. He was pleased with managing to complete the paperwork and informed Brett that Sam's admission was complete without highlighting the issues about Sam's recent stress and the disruption to his eating pattern.

Activity 2.1   Critical thinking

In the case study above, what might be the repercussions for Graham, Brett and Sam of failing to report the issue of Sam's stress and disrupted eating in the patient assessment? How does this scenario relate to the 6Cs?

An outline answer is given at the end of the chapter.

As the case study highlights, assessment undertaken with – rather than on – patients is preferable because an inclusive approach is more likely to gain patient cooperation and more accurate information. Not only that, but the planned outcomes it elicits are more likely to align with what the patient actually wants. Such an assessment is called person-centred because not only does it take account of the patient's wishes, but it also takes account of the patient's lifeworld. This means all the elements that make up the patient's everyday life, including relevant family/friends, daily activities, preferences and interests. In their research into trust in the pre-hospital non-urgent care setting, Norberg Boysen et al. (2017) identify how attention to the lifeworld of the patient by healthcare professionals contributes to the patient having trust in the professional and the care environment; something which, contrary to what many nurses believe, is not automatically granted in many care interactions.

As the case study highlights, adding the information about Sam's recent stress and eating pattern might enable a broader assessment of his needs and more focused use of resources. The purpose of assessment is to identify what treatment, services or care the patient needs, but more importantly whether the patient also wants them (Field and Smith, 2008). Graham's response suggests he is focused on the task of admitting Sam and completing the documentation rather than listening attentively to what Sam is saying. We now proceed to look at the nurse's role in patient assessment.

What is the nurse's role in patient assessment?

Undertaking a patient assessment requires the nurse to draw on different forms of knowledge. Carper (1978) defined the 'ways of knowing' required in nursing as *empirics, aesthetics* and *ethics* (page 14). In essence, what this means is that evidence-based knowledge (empirics) should be used to underpin patient assessment, but that employing caring behaviours to help build a therapeutic relationship (aesthetics) with your patient is of equal importance and also needs to be underpinned by ethical behaviour. The Royal College of Nursing has acknowledged that trying to define the knowledge that nurses use is complex and not necessarily helpful, as nursing is constantly evolving (RCN, 2003). In 2009, Moule and Goodman (page 15) defined nursing knowledge as being 'drawn from a multifaceted base' and including 'evidence that comes from science (research and evaluation), experience and personally derived understanding'.

A more recent definition of nursing knowledge suggests:

> *Nursing knowledge is characterized by diverse and multiple forms of knowing and underpins the work of all nurses, regardless of field of practice.*
>
> (Sakamoto, 2018, e12209)

From this perspective, nursing knowledge stems from implementing both theory and practice, including psychosocial and cultural elements as well as practical processes. One of the dangers of applying simplistic holism, that is holistic practice which does not account for the variety of ways of knowing, is that nurses limit their perceptions and understanding of practice (Stiles, 2011) and in so doing limit the offer of care available to the patient. As a nursing process, therefore, patient assessment also draws on the expertise of the nurse in being able to evaluate what is helpful, and what is less so, within the assessment process. Reflecting on such processes helps to add to your knowledge base and develop your practice as a professional.

It is important for you to clarify the focus of the assessment in order for patients to be able to respond appropriately. This requires you to start from a position of understanding your own feelings about the assessment and the patient, as these can influence the assessment process and be revealed by your body language. The following case study offers an example of a nurse needing to control her own feelings when assessing the needs of a patient.

Case study: Vanessa's child assessment

Vanessa was in the first year of her child nursing training. She was working with her practice supervisor, Meena, on a children's ward in an acute hospital. Vanessa had previously been shown how to carry out an initial admission assessment, and so was completing the assessment under supervision today.

(Continued)

(Continued)

Emily was 5 years old and was being admitted from accident and emergency (A&E) with a broken arm following a fall from her bicycle. The A&E nurse told Meena and Vanessa privately that there was some suspicion that the fall might not have been accidental. Vanessa began the assessment by checking how Emily was feeling. However, Vanessa found it difficult to maintain eye contact with Emily's mother when she was asking her the assessment questions. Emily's mother responded by giving short answers. A few times Meena had to intervene to find out more information. Afterwards, Meena discussed with Vanessa how she thought the assessment had gone. Vanessa said she felt that she had got the relevant information but found it difficult to talk to the mother because of thinking how Emily might have broken her arm. Meena explained how she had observed Vanessa's non-verbal communication betraying her judgement of Emily's mother, which affected the responses the mother was making, and therefore the quality of the patient assessment. Meena emphasised the need to suppress our personal feelings in order to get the necessary information and to give unbiased care. Vanessa acknowledged that she found this a hard lesson to learn.

The case study above illustrates how personal feelings can sometimes cloud our judgement and why it is important first of all to master our own feelings and behaviours. Completing Activity 2.2 will help you to examine your own feelings about some of the different patients you might encounter.

Activity 2.2   Reflection

Make a list of situations where you have found it difficult to provide unbiased care for a patient, or to talk to a member of their family or someone accompanying them. Now reflect on why you found it difficult to care for them. What does the code of professional standards of practice and behaviour for nurses, midwives and nursing associates say a nurse must do in such circumstances (see the NMC weblink at the end of the chapter)?

Which of the 6Cs is most relevant and absent in your experiences and in the case study above?

Although this activity is based on your own experience, there is a limited answer at the end of the chapter.

Your experiences, or those of people close to you, are likely to have influenced the list you made. For example, you might have included those who perpetrate domestic violence or other abuses. Being aware of your reactions is an important first step to being able to deal with them, especially as in many cases our original suspicions about someone may turn out to be wrong. Having the 6Cs at the forefront of your thinking, and being aware of the code of professional standards of practice and behaviour for nurses, midwives and nursing associates (NMC, 2018b) can help you to reflect on your reactions and to respond positively.

If you have a number of patients to care for, you will also need to prioritise whose assessment is the most clinically important (Sully and Dallas, 2010) rather than reacting according to your own biases or prejudices or making snap moral judgements (Hill, 2010). There are ethical elements to prioritisation, and failure to get it right can be detrimental to the patient and cause the nurse moral distress (Suhonen et al., 2018). Nurses do need to make judgements about care needs, but should not make judgements about people, as these can be based on assumption, and therefore skew the accuracy of the patient assessment. The nurse's role in patient assessment is to work with patients to identify their nursing needs and preferences and to gather information on behalf of other professionals involved in the patient's care.

Why is accurate patient assessment so important?

Accurate patient assessment is important in order to plan appropriate care that meets the patient's needs. To be able to carry out an accurate patient assessment, you may also need to employ assessment tools (e.g. a wound assessment tool or a pressure area scoring system). Such tools enable the nurse to integrate important subjective information with objective data to produce a more accurate and reliable profile of the patient's needs. You can read more about how to use subjective and objective information in Chapter 3 and about assessment tools in Chapter 4. The following case study illustrates why accurate patient assessment is so important.

Case study: Mustafa's assessment

Mustafa is 88 years old and has recently lost mobility. He is cared for by his daughter at home. After a recent fall, he has lost confidence and wants to stay mainly in bed. As a result, he has developed a pressure sore on his sacrum. The district nurse, Katarina, is looking after him. Katarina has a holiday booked in the next week and Mustafa's daughter has noticed him becoming agitated.

Katarina is keen to ensure that her colleagues who are going to look after Mustafa maintain the same regimen, as she knows he does not like change. She is therefore careful to document the pressure ulcer score and any contributing factors, as well as the wound dressing used. To aid with assessment, she also takes a photograph – with Mustafa's consent – so that all the assessment data can be reviewed subjectively and objectively.

(Continued)

(Continued)

Mustafa does not respond well to Gabby, Katarina's replacement, often refusing to cooperate. She calls another nurse, Fatima, to help out. Fatima changes the pressure ulcer dressing after three days and notes that it appears to look better. She is basing this on visual inspection. She documents the improvement and tells Mustafa, who is pleased.

When Katarina is back from her holiday, the first thing Mustafa tells her is of the improvement in his pressure sore. When she inspects it and compares it to the photo she took, Katarina notes that it has in fact enlarged at one edge. She is left with the dilemma of what to say to Mustafa without compromising her colleague.

The case study highlights that it is important to be able to assess changes objectively and accurately, where this is possible, in order to provide appropriate treatment and accurate information, as well as document the care planning process. When Fatima assessed Mustafa, the assessment was incomplete because she had based it on her subjective opinion and not included more objective information, such as that provided by the photo of the wound. Therefore, while the wound may have appeared to be getting better, the information about this that she gave to Mustafa was inaccurate. Any wound assessment needs to encompass wound bed condition as well as wound size and other factors such as the presence of slough or granulating tissue. What makes an assessment good is making sure the information collected is complete and, as far as possible, objective. This may involve other professionals who may have a different view of the assessment required but whose input to the overall evaluation of the problem is important (Kara et al., 2018). Completing Activity 2.3 will help you to identify what other professionals might be involved in Mustafa's care and how these individuals might contribute to a more holistic overall assessment.

Activity 2.3   Critical thinking

When thinking about Mustafa's case, who else do you think might be involved in his care and what would they be assessing in particular? Ask your practice supervisor who the tissue viability nurse is in your placement area and ask that individual what assessment strategies they use.

Which of the 6Cs is most relevant to Mustafa's case and why?

An outline answer is given at the end of the chapter.

Completing this activity should not only help you to identify other relevant professionals involved in Mustafa's care, but also demonstrate the importance of integrating their different perspectives before planning care. One review of the literature relating to interprofessional collaboration in the care of older patients (Tsakitzidis et al., 2016) identified among its benefits:

- increased professional satisfaction;
- increased patient satisfaction;
- improved quality of healthcare; and
- reduced mortality.

It is important for patients to experience a seamless service if they are to be confident that their needs are being properly assessed and communicated. In Mustafa's case, this means using validated standardised approaches to wound assessment or treatment, as well as using the objective data available from the photograph. Most health and social care organisations have adopted specific tools that are incorporated into their patient assessment documentation. Such tools are usually generated based on research, which in turn informs both guidelines and organisational policy. Wound assessment charts vary between organisations, but commonly consider the dimensions of the wound, the appearance of the wound bed and surrounding skin, any exudate or bleeding, the level of pain, and the location of the wound to be entered on the body map (Dougherty et al., 2015). The case study highlights that professionals need to be honest about any gaps in their understanding and explain to patients why they are pursuing certain avenues of enquiry, because our ways of knowing vary.

Four ways of working with facts

Healthcare practice is uncertain because we are dealing with unique individuals who do not always respond in the ways we expect. It is important for health practitioners to be able to deal with this uncertainty constructively in order for patients to be able to trust them. When we are working, we usually access our knowledge to try to make decisions about what to do. Girard (2007) identifies four ways of knowing. How this relates to dealing with facts is set out in Table 2.1 using Johari window principles to consider areas that are known, others we are currently blind to, some we have not yet discovered, and others we are unaware of (Luft and Ingham, 1955, cited in Hillson and Murray-Webster, 2007, page 116).

Facts you know you know	Facts you know you don't know
Available information that you can use (e.g. the name and age of the patient and the patient's problem)	Gaps in the information, where you know you need to find out more (e.g. what medication the patient takes/whether the patient has any allergies)
Facts you know but don't know that you know	**Facts you don't know you don't know**
Knowledge you have but are not aware of until it is needed (e.g. how to deal with a fire)	Information you are not aware that you need and need to discover (e.g. what to do about a patient's non-compliance)

Table 2.1 Four areas of factual knowledge

Being able to identify the four areas of factual knowledge is an important step to understanding how you think and how you can tap into knowledge that you might not know you have. Read the following case study and then complete Activity 2.4 in order to find out what you currently know and don't know, and more importantly what else you need to know to understand patients' needs and give effective care.

Case study: Mr Haughton's admission

Mr Haughton is a 60-year-old man with leukaemia. He is admitted to the ward with pyrexia of 38.6°C and nausea. He had a laparoscopic cholecystectomy two months previously. Mr Haughton has blood taken and an abdominal X-ray is done. He is started on IV fluids and antibiotics. After ten days in hospital, Mr Haughton is able to return home.

Activity 2.4   Reflection

Review Mr Haughton's case and try to identify how your knowledge fits into the four areas illustrated in Table 2.1.

An outline answer is given at the end of the chapter.

Mr Haughton's case highlights that patients may have a number of concurrent problems, and this makes assessing and caring for them complex. While you may have knowledge about some of these, there are also areas that you need to discover more about. You may also need to understand how different problems interact with each other. Understanding that there are always gaps in our knowledge and that we need to be aware of areas we are ignorant of is an important aspect of understanding yourself in the assessment process and what you need to do. You might identify that you lack knowledge about the patient's condition or what decision to make. You might want to include others, such as your practice supervisor or another professional, in your thinking and decision-making processes. Standing's (2023) cognitive continuum might offer some ideas regarding how we think about making decisions in practice (for more information on making decisions within patient assessment, see Chapter 9).

Standing's cognitive continuum and relevance to nurses and patient assessment

Making decisions when assessing patients means understanding the evidence base for practice. There are a number of modes of practice according to Standing (2023, page 8). These are:

- intuitive judgement – sensing patient concerns and changes;
- reflective judgement – moment-by-moment reviewing and revising of your practice;
- patient and peer-aided judgement – reaching consensus decisions with the patient and others;
- system-aided judgement – making use of policies and assessment tools;
- critical review of experience and research evidence – critical evaluation of your experience and available research that underpins this;
- action research and clinical audit – evaluating practice against benchmarks;
- qualitative research – interpreting the patient experience;
- survey research – making use of trends of evidence within particular populations; and
- experimental research – identifying generalisable evidence.

It is important for you to know what evidence you are drawing upon within patient assessment and care planning in order to ensure that you can justify the decisions you make to the patient and to the profession. This will be discussed further in Chapter 9, but we begin here with a case study and an activity to help you critically consider your current knowledge and skills.

Case study: Lily's bowel problem

Lily is 45 years old and has recently been having problems with urgency and faecal incontinence. She has seen her GP, who has diagnosed irritable bowel syndrome, and as part of her care refers Lily to the specialist bladder and bowel nurse, Nicky. At Lily's assessment, Nicky takes a full history and asks Lily to keep a diary of her dietary and fluid intake and bladder and bowel actions. She also completes a bladder scan, which is normal. Nicky asks Lily to look at the Bristol stool chart and identify which best matches her normal stool appearance. Lily identifies that her stools best match types 4 and 5, which are smooth and soft, sometimes too soft. Nicky advises Lily that she needs to cut down on her fruit intake and explains ways for Lily to manage her occasional faecal incontinence. Nicky makes an appointment to see Lily again in six weeks.

In the case study, Nicky, the specialist bladder and bowel nurse, has gathered her evidence through talking to Lily about her history and eating habits, identified precisely the type of stool Lily is producing, excluded a bladder problem via the scan, and used her knowledge of research and practice to advise Lily on a plan of action. When completing an assessment, if we simply said to patients, 'You need to stop eating so much fruit', they would understandably be reluctant unless we can provide the evidence for our recommendation. Completing Activity 2.5 will help you to explore how you might use the different modes in your own practice.

Activity 2.5 Reflection

Think about your last placement and the different patients you nursed. Consider in what circumstances you can identify using a particular mode from Standing's (2023) continuum. Why was this mode of practice particularly relevant to the situation?

Although this activity is based on your own experience, there is a limited answer at the end of the chapter.

You might have made a system-aided judgement by using an assessment tool to help gain further information, or reflective judgement adapting how you were communicating as you talked with the patient. Less obvious is how we add all the understandings from the modes of practice together to come to the decisions we do. It is important to understand these thinking processes ourselves so we can explain them to the patient (as we saw Nicky do) and to other health professionals to justify the courses of action we propose. Given reasonable and well-presented evidence, patients might be more informed, and therefore more inclined to engage in the assessment and subsequent treatment processes. That said, it is important to recognise the subjective nature of truth in terms of what patients tell us and what we think is important. Completing Activity 2.6 will help you to understand that the truth we are seeking in patient assessment is what patients' needs are and the most effective way to help them.

Activity 2.6 Reflection

Reflect on what various forms of evidence you might need to undertake an assessment of a patient and plan their subsequent care.

An outline answer is given at the end of the chapter.

How we put together the narratives patients give us with the other facets of our information-gathering within the context of our practice knowledge and policy is complex. Much of our initial assessment will be based on what the patient is reporting, but they may not understand that a minor symptom to them could aid in assessment of their care needs. The following case study will illustrate this point.

The nature of truth

Case study: Lucy's pain experience

Lucy was a woman with learning disabilities living in an assisted living setting. She complained of stomach cramps during her normal menstruation and was usually given paracetamol by the support workers. Lucy was admitted to the local hospital for a minor procedure. A carer came with her but could not stay all the time. Lucy became distressed when she was in pain. The staff on the ward tried to calm her but Lucy got more and more distressed. Lucy was given pain medication, but not as frequently as she could have it, as the staff assumed that her agitation was part of her normal behaviour. The assessment tool they used for assessing pain was validated for use with children. Lucy was left unnecessarily in pain because the staff did not believe her and had made assumptions about her.

What Lucy's case study highlights is that we may use our own pain experience or behavioural norms to interpret the experiences of others rather than accepting the truth taken from their perspective. In doing so, we may use stereotyping assumptions for interpretation. McCaffery (1968) famously stated that 'pain is whatever the experiencing person says it is, existing whenever the experiencing person says it does' (page 95); this highlights the issue that people both experience and express pain in different ways. The role of the nurse is to accept this definition without being judgemental or applying our own preconceived ideas as to what pain is or is not.

The case study illustrates a failure to live by three elements of the 6Cs: communication, care and competence. The nurses failed to communicate meaningfully with Lucy, they failed to provide adequate pain relief, which is a failure in care, and they demonstrated a lack of competence in understanding pain from her point of view.

Truth is determined by ourselves in accordance with our values and beliefs, by others and how influential we perceive them to be, and by society as a whole. For example, those perceived to be in a powerful position, such as doctors, may not be questioned about their version of the truth. In mental health nursing, we might call into question the singular nature of reality when many patients experience something very different. Therefore, truth remains tentative and uncertain and subjective in nature. Sometimes when truth is perceived to be what is expressed by another, the subjective view is discounted, closing down the ability to look at personal experience (Frosh, 2002). What this means is that if professionals impose their interpretation of the patient's experience on to the patient, it is less likely that patients will be able to tell what their actual experience is, and they may just go along with what the professional suggests. Decisions based on such a flawed perspective will then be compromised and may fail to be in the patient's best interests (however the patient defines these).

Stereotyping

Stereotyping is a way of categorising things and people that allows us to draw on previous experiences of those categories to direct our actions, which is quicker than forming new categories (Goodman and Clemow, 2010). That is to say we put people into categories (or boxes) according to our previous experiences, or assumed prejudices, of people we perceive as being similar to them. The negative effect of stereotyping is making assumptions about another person that are unlikely to be accurate. We stereotype based on our personal values, beliefs and experiences, and this may relate to patients, colleagues and peers. For example, if we saw a man weaving along the street looking dishevelled, we might stereotype him as being drunk, even though there are many reasons why someone might be moving in that way (e.g. they may have multiple sclerosis, be experiencing a diabetic hypoglycaemic episode or have sustained a head injury). As highlighted in the case study of Lucy, stereotyping can equally cause us to make inaccurate assumptions about why someone is behaving in a particular way. If a health or social care professional is working from such an assumption, patient assessment will not only be affected, but it could be wildly inaccurate and dangerous. Completing Activity 2.7 will help you to examine situations where you may have been stereotyping people.

Activity 2.7 Reflection

Think about a recent practice experience where you think you, or someone else, might have been stereotyping someone and consider the following questions:

1. Why do you think that person was stereotyped?
2. What was the result of stereotyping that individual?
3. What experiences might have led to the stereotyping of this person?

As this activity is based on your personal experience, there is no outline answer at the end of the chapter.

You might be stereotyping by using norms for situations, such as how to behave in class or in the professional setting, and expectations of particular roles (Goodman and Clemow, 2010). You might assume that someone is suffering from a particular condition because you have seen something similar before – this is itself a form of stereotyping as we are drawing on our 'previous experiences of those categories' to direct our thinking. Such stereotyping, or perhaps more correctly categorisation, is not always a bad thing: it enables professionals to respond quickly and assuredly in an emergency situation, for example. However, if stereotyping results in diminishing someone else's choices, the effects are not helpful. We need to consider our own values and responses and adjust our professional behaviour.

Conclusion

Good patient assessment is the goal for the nurse because in order to provide good care, we need to learn a lot about our patients. We can only do this by accessing and applying the full range of relevant evidence at our disposal. This process of gathering and responding to the collected knowledge is what is known as an inductive process; that is, a process in which the nurse allows the evidence to guide them to a conclusion rather than forming a conclusion and looking for the evidence to support it – sometimes called deductive reasoning (Creswell and Poth, 2017). Nevertheless, it is also recognised that nurses and patients are individuals who have their own values and ideas which need to be reconciled in order for accurate patient assessment and care planning to ensue. This may sometimes be difficult to do, but in the process we can learn a lot about ourselves and become better professionals.

Chapter summary

This chapter has clarified what patient assessment is and why it is important. It has identified some factors that are helpful and some that are hindering to effective patient assessment, looking in particular at the influence of personal values and attitudes and application of the 6Cs. The activities included have invited you to consider your own values as you need to grasp how influential these are when you are assessing a patient. The chapter has also introduced Standing's (2023) nine modes of practice as a way of thinking about how you justify your thought processes and the decisions that you make. This will be discussed further in Chapter 9.

Activities: brief outline answers

Activity 2.1   Critical thinking (page 24)

Graham has not thought through the implications of Sam's strict veganism and how this might affect his diabetes at a time of high stress. A further dietitian referral might be needed, or it might not, depending on what actually caused the hypoglycaemic episodes. Brett is accountable for this gap, and by not following up the information, his mistake could result in Sam being at further risk of poor management of his diabetes when he leaves the hospital. Sam's knowledge about how to manage his diabetes remains compromised due to his dietetic and stress management needs not being adequately explored by Graham. This case study highlights how important commitment – one of the 6Cs – to the person is, and not just the task being completed.

Activity 2.2   Reflection (page 26)

You might have included the following within your list:

- drunk driver;
- drug addict;

- paedophile;
- rapist;
- murderer; and/or
- terrorist.

The code of professional standards of practice and behaviour for nurses, midwives and nursing associates (NMC, 2018b) is clear that all nurses must treat people as individuals. This means you must:

- treat all people with kindness, respect and compassion;
- avoid making assumptions and recognise diversity and individual choice;
- act with honesty and integrity at all times, treating people fairly and without discrimination, bullying or harassment; and
- be aware at all times of how your behaviour can affect and influence the behaviour of other people.

Compassion – one of the 6Cs – is the most relevant here because it demonstrates drawing alongside someone and not judging them, but trying to discern their needs.

Activity 2.3   Critical thinking (page 28)

The other people involved in Mustafa's care are likely to include his GP, who will be overseeing the progress of healing of his pressure ulcer. Mustafa may also be assessed by a dietitian, who will be evaluating his nutritional needs and preferences. Mustafa could also be assessed by the specialist tissue viability nurse, who will be monitoring the wound and healing specifically and offering advice on wound dressing options. A multidisciplinary meeting would help to integrate these assessment processes, but in the community setting comprehensive integrated notes are more often used for this purpose. Competence – one of the 6Cs – is the most relevant to this case in terms of how Fatima assessed Mustafa's pressure ulcer. Of course one element of Mustafa's care which may need to be re-addressed is his fear of falling and there may be good reasons to refer him to the community physiotherapy team to help get him on his feet again.

Activity 2.4   Reflection (page 30)

The facts you know are Mr Haughton's age, the conditions he has come in with, his history of a laparoscopic cholecystectomy, and that he is pyrexial. The facts you know you don't know are his normal medication, any allergies, what type of leukaemia he has and how it is normally treated, and whether the pyrexia is due to his leukaemia or something going on with his previous surgery. The facts you don't know you know are about blood components and what they do, and you can therefore link this to how Mr Haughton is likely to be affected by his leukaemia. The facts you don't know you don't know are likely to be related to Mr Haughton's healing response in the light of having leukaemia and any other aspects of his condition or care that you have not thought about.

Activity 2.5   Reflection (page 32)

You are likely to have used intuitive judgement such as realising that the patient was upset when you made your assessment and trying to understand the patient's response. At the same time, you are likely to have reflected on your own communication – one of the 6Cs – with the patient and how perhaps your tone of voice allowed that person to open up to you. You will have needed to interpret the patient's experience from what he or she told you. You may have needed to consult with your practice supervisor about the assessment or care planning process, as well as checking whether the patient was in agreement with what you planned. Using an assessment tool such as the Bristol stool chart might have helped you to collect accurate details on which to base your clinical judgement. When evaluating your practice experience more broadly, such as for your portfolio, you may have considered how your practice fits with the NMC Standards and the 6Cs and what you are actually using to underpin what you do.

Activity 2.6   Reflection (page 32)

You might have included:

- the story/history that the patient gives about a need or problem;
- nursing observations;
- assessment tool results;
- peer-aided judgements such as discussion with your practice supervisor or multidisciplinary meeting outcomes;
- research findings; and/or
- policies and guidelines.

Further reading

Goodman, B and Clemow, R (2010) *Nursing and Collaborative Practice: A Guide to Interprofessional Learning and Working* (2nd edn). Exeter: Learning Matters.

A useful book for understanding how professionals' values can influence their approach to patients and each other and guidance on how to work more collaboratively.

Standing, M (2023) *Clinical Judgement and Decision-Making in Nursing* (5th edn). London: SAGE.

This book introduces decision-making theory and its relevance to nursing practice.

Useful website

www.nmc-uk.org

The website of the Nursing and Midwifery Council, where you can find a great deal of professional information, including the latest guidance on the code of professional standards of practice and behaviour for nurses, midwives and nursing associates.

Chapter 3 Making sense of patient information

Peter Ellis

Platform 4: Providing and evaluating care

At the point of registration, the registered nurse will be able to:

4.2   work in partnership with people to encourage shared decision making in order to support individuals, their families and carers to manage their own care when appropriate.

4.3   demonstrate the knowledge, communication and relationship management skills required to provide people, families and carers with accurate information that meets their needs before, during and after a range of interventions.

Chapter aims

After reading this chapter, you will be able to:

* differentiate between different types and forms of information;
* identify different ways of gathering information;
* differentiate between the nurse's and other professionals' roles in gathering patient information;
* identify when and why gathering information could be challenging;
* understand how to prioritise nursing actions from the information gained during assessment; and
* make sense of the information received from patients through checking accuracy of understanding, and be able to interpret and explain this to others.

Introduction

Case study: James's recent hospital visit

James is 68 years old and has been admitted to hospital for a number of conditions over the last few years. He is brought to your placement ward complaining of pain in his upper abdomen. James has quite a thick file of notes from his previous investigations and admissions. In the emergency department, James has had blood taken, an electrocardiogram (ECG), and baseline pulse, temperature, blood pressure and oxygen saturations. Your practice supervisor, Tamara, suggests you talk to James to find out how he is feeling and what he understands as being the problem. Tamara also asks you to repeat the nursing observations while she checks through the notes for his history and the computer for his blood results. James tells you that he has previously had an oesophageal gastroduodenoscopy (OGD),

(Continued)

(Continued)

and this found a small ulcer, which he thinks might be what is causing him pain. He also tells you that he recently retired and has been drinking a bit more than usual because he feels so low. Your practice supervisor tells you that his blood count indicates that he is anaemic, which might suggest that he is bleeding from somewhere. His ECG is normal, however.

When you complete James's nursing observations, you note he is a little tachycardic, which could also mean he is bleeding from somewhere. Subsequently, James has a further OGD, which demonstrates the ulcer has enlarged and is bleeding. Following a blood transfusion, James's medication is increased, and he is advised to cut down his alcohol intake and is discharged home. In order to help James manage his feeling of isolation following retirement, the ward social worker refers him to a retirees support group.

No matter how long or short their history, a great variety of information is gathered from patients when they enter the health and social care setting. As the above case study identifies, this information needs to be interpreted swiftly and accurately. What is also of note here for the nurse seeking to undertake a holistic assessment is the interplay between James's personal circumstances and his health issues. It is part of the nurse's role to make sense of this diversity of information by checking with the patient and others, and to use the information obtained accurately in planning appropriate care *with* the patient. In the above case study, the nurse checks with James what his view of the problem is, and the accuracy of the history found in the notes, then she integrates this with nursing observations and test results. As a student, you need to be able to gather relevant patient information and interpret it by identifying its meaning and significance and referring to other health professionals. This is important for developing your communication competence with others.

This chapter starts by defining patient information, establishing the roles of different healthcare professionals in gathering patient information. The chapter categorises different forms of information, identifying the strengths and weaknesses of these categories. It goes on to consider the appropriateness of different approaches to questioning, such as the use of open, closed, probing and laddering questions. A variety of activities are offered to encourage you to make sense of information, identify situations where gathering information is difficult, differentiate the role of the nurse from that of other healthcare professionals, and learn how to analyse information and use the analysis in order to act on it. Throughout these activities, you will be asked to reflect on the patient assessment process.

What is patient information?

Patient information is any information that relates to a patient. This will include personal details, such as name, age and date of birth, as well as information relating to the individual's social and medical history and current health status. It is gathered by health and social care professionals for the purpose of helping the patient. Different fields of practice focus on different aspects of information and gather elements of the information offered in different amounts of depth. For example, mental health nurses may be concerned more with the psychosocial information about a patient than their general nurse colleagues. For the mental health team, therefore, information relating to family history, behaviour, mood, mental state, recreational activities and relationships is all deemed particularly relevant and important. Occupational therapy is concerned with what individuals can do for themselves in relation to the activities of daily living, while physiotherapists focus upon information relating to mobility and physical activity. Both professional groups, occupational therapists and physiotherapists, are interested in gathering information to support rehabilitating the patient. Therefore, patient capabilities and preferences are the main focus. Social work considers the social context in which the individual lives, particularly in relation to vulnerability.

Medicine is concerned with identifying and solving medical problems, an approach that has been described as taking a *deficit view*. Increasingly, doctors now take part in health promotion activities as well. Because of nurses' unique position of being in close and regular contact with patients, they are able to coordinate making sense of information with patients, interpreting terms, and explaining things patients do not understand. This includes listening to the patient and picking up on information others may not have gathered as well as observing for signs which may be missed by other professionals who visit the patient infrequently, e.g. a grimace which might indicate pain. This offers the opportunity for achieving a more *holistic* perspective, which takes account of the patient's views as well as integrating a variety of professional opinions, as appropriate. 'Holistic' means a complete view that involves the patient. We now proceed to consider different types and forms of patient information. For further reading on what information is gathered in different settings of care, see Howatson-Jones and Ellis (2008).

Different types and forms of information

In its simplest form, information can be divided into *subjective* and *objective* information. This can also be related to intuitive forms of thinking versus more rational and analytical forms of assessment (Standing, 2023). For example, in the case study about James Ashton, objective information has been obtained from the nursing observations, the ECG and the blood results, which give a physiological view of the problem. Equally important, however, is the subjective information that James has conveyed about how he is feeling and what he perceives the problem to be. Through this line of questioning, other important information about his low mood and increased drinking is discovered. This case study highlights the importance of using both types of information in order to interpret accurately what is really happening.

Subjective information relates to the descriptions patients give of their experience and understanding of the situation. Your interpretation skills add another form of subjective information based on your professional experience. For example, when a patient describes a pain experience, you will be observing their non-verbal behaviour as well as listening to the description. It is likely you will also be filtering your interpretation of the patient's pain experience through your *intuitive* knowledge of what is going on.

The weakness of relying solely on subjective information is that it is based on particular experience, interpreted through the lens of the experience you have had, and as a result you may miss other important cues of what is going on. Objective information is mostly *quantitative* data (data that can be measured, e.g. vital signs such as pulse and blood pressure and tests such as blood test results, which list the levels of different blood cells and electrolytes). The weakness of relying solely on objective information is that it signals an alteration has taken place but does not identify why this may have happened or how this affects the person. Objective information gathering also often fails to identify symptoms which are subjective and relate to what the person is feeling and experiencing. These can only be understood through asking, although some tools (such as pain scales) exist, which try to help objectify symptoms.

Activity 3.1   Reflection

Reflect on the case study about James Ashton. Consider how the information gathered in the patient assessment was both objective and subjective.

Consider how these different forms of information were subsequently used to inform the interventions offered to James. What might have happened if not all of the forms of information had been collected?

An outline answer is given at the end of the chapter.

The main types of information gathered from patients and potential sources are given in Table 3.1, although this list is not exhaustive.

Subjective and objective information may also appear in different forms:

- repeated information – this often comes from family and friends or carers who reinforce and help to elaborate the patient's story (e.g. what tests the patient has had and what they have been told);
- observation – this information is gathered by closely observing the patient (e.g. being aware of the quality of the patient's breathing, how the patient is moving, and the patient's mood); and
- clinical information – this emerges from clinical activity with the patient (e.g. recording observations, doing a wound dressing, and checking pressure areas).

A good patient assessment involves gathering a mix of both forms of information and using your senses: your eyes to observe patient behaviours, movement and how the patient looks; your ears to listen to breathing and what the patient is really saying; your touch to feel what is revealed by the skin; and your smell to detect odours (Howatson-Jones and Ellis, 2008). This information remains subjective (i.e. open to individual interpretation) and is also reliant on nursing experience, and is therefore very individual. Integrating objective information in order to confirm or deny the conclusions drawn from the collection and interpretation of subjective data is therefore important. For this reason, when checking someone's pressure areas, you will use your visual observations as well as the more objective Waterlow screening tool in order to assess for risk factors you cannot see. The following two case studies illustrate what can happen if health professionals do not integrate the subjective with the objective, but focus on one aspect only. Inexperience can result in unrealistic solutions.

Subjective	Part subjective, part objective	Objective
Biographical details – usually sourced from the patient themself, but if they are incapacitated in some way information may be obtained from family/friends/carers or from documentary evidence, and relate not only to what the person can actually remember, but also their interpretation of this.	Medical history – a chronological sequence of events taken by a doctor, which integrates relevant test results with physical examination. Usually uses a biomedical focus on the problem (for the type of information sought, see **www. gpnotebook.co.uk**). Again, in the absence of pre-existing notes, this is affected by memory and interpretation.	Test results – sourced from diagnostic and interventional techniques that examine anatomical and physiological activity within narrow margins of normal and abnormal. These have usually developed from clinical trials – the highest level of research evidence (Ellis, 2023). Test modalities and retrieval involve technology requiring healthcare professionals to be health informatics-literate to access and process results (Hutchfield, 2010).
Social context – usually sourced from the patient, but often added to by family/friends/carers and by healthcare professional assessments, such as occupational therapist, social worker community nursing and care managers.	Referral information – sourced from a variety of healthcare professionals, including general practitioners, specialist doctors/nurses, occupational therapists, physiotherapists, mental health teams, social workers, care managers, speech therapists and dieticians, and will also include any relevant test and observation results.	

(Continued)

Table 3.1   (Continued)

Subjective	Part subjective, part objective	Objective
Symptoms – sourced from the patient but may be added to by family/ friends/carers (see **www. patients.uptodate.com**).	Prescription – sourced from general practitioner/patient/ family/carer. Pharmacist will review before dispensing.	
Observations – sourced from a variety of healthcare professionals, including nurses, occupational therapists, physiotherapists, dietitians, doctors and others.		

Table 3.1   Types of information and potential sources

Case study: Mrs Harrison's diabetic control

Mrs Harrison lives with Type 2 diabetes, for which she takes tablets. She mostly manages this herself at home, but her practice nurse has called her for a regular review at the surgery. A blood test is taken for glycosylated haemoglobin. This is a test that measures the amount of glucose bound to haemoglobin, and can be an accurate measure of the average levels of blood glucose in the preceding three months, and therefore the level of glucose control. The result came back as 89mmol/mol, which is significantly raised. The National Institute for Health and Care Excellence (NICE, 2022) recommend that most adults living with diabetes aim for a level of 4.8mmol/mol. No one was aware that during this time, Mrs Harrison's husband had left her. The stress of this is likely to have contributed to the raised blood glucose levels through the release of glucocorticoids, which are hormones released by stress. While the interventions chosen might be relevant, they do not address the main problem, which is Mrs Harrison's stress level.

Case study: Angelina's adaptation needs

Angelina is in her seventies and lives alone at home. She has been having difficulty getting about and washing and is generally finding it harder to manage. She is visited by Monika, a community team occupational therapist, who is relatively new. Angelina tells Monika what she would like. Monika completes her patient assessment and identifies that Angelina requires a number of aids and alterations to help her continue to live a relatively independent life.

Her recommendations are for grab handrails to be fitted, for the bathroom to be converted into a wet room shower, and for a stairlift to be installed. Angelina is delighted with these proposals. However, Angelina is less happy when Monika returns the following week to say that perhaps they need to start by trying out some handrails on the stairs first and look at other ways of helping Angelina with washing. Monika's lack of experience meant that her subjective view of the situation was unrealistic and she set up expectations which could not be met.

As demonstrated in the two case studies, focusing on the subjective and objective separately means that important patient information is missed and is not considered in planning interventions. They also demonstrate the importance of working with patients and their carers (if relevant), and not planning care from a purely professional viewpoint. We now proceed to consider when patients should be assessed.

When to assess patients

Patients need to be assessed at key points in their care journey. It is important to assess patients when they first identify they have a need, when meeting them for the first time, when their needs change, and when accepting, referring or discharging them. Where different healthcare practitioners are involved, it may also be necessary to complete different assessments, although increasingly healthcare teams are becoming integrated. This is particularly true of the interface between acute and community care, where the purpose of integrated teams is to reduce the assessment burden on the patient and promote a seamless service. Therefore, it may be possible that a therapist or a nurse undertakes some of the patient assessments. Situations that can make patient assessment difficult are those where the patient is not capable of responding or where patient response is impaired in some way. Completing Activity 3.2 will help you to think about some situations where this could be the case.

Activity 3.2   Critical thinking

What situations might make gathering information from the patient difficult, and what other methods might you use instead? To help you complete this activity, think back to your most recent placement experiences.

An outline answer is given at the end of the chapter.

We now proceed to consider some questioning techniques when gathering patient information.

Questioning techniques

Gaining a good rapport with a patient is an important part of creating the environment in which to gather the information needed to make a nursing diagnosis. This process also requires the nurse to develop a good questioning technique so that the patient can understand what is being asked and for the health professional to gain, in a complete and structured way, the information required to inform diagnostic and therapeutic processes.

It is imperative to build a good therapeutic relationship and trust before launching into questioning. Egan (2014) identifies that important communication skills, such as attentive listening, being open, responding and reflecting, are needed to help people tell their story and to develop dialogue that gets to the core of the matter through probing, and which aids understanding through summarising (Grant and Goodman, 2018). The way you respond to a patient the first time you meet that person sets the tone for the rest of the encounter, and is therefore crucial to establishing trust and subsequent dialogue. Take some time to complete Activity 3.3 and reflect on your communication with new patients.

Activity 3.3   Reflection

Reflect on previous encounters you have had with new patients and consider the following questions:

1. What went well and what did not go so well?
2. Why might this have been?
3. What strategies have you already developed to improve your rapport with patients?
4. How can you help patients who have difficulty in supplying information?

As this activity is based on your experience, there is no outline answer at the end of the chapter.

Reflecting on your own patient encounters may have highlighted that it is not always easy to elicit information and relying on your current communication skills may not be enough. If you have not had much experience in practice, the following case study may help you to consider some of the issues involved in communicating with patients.

Case study: Johann's questioning experience

Johann was on a placement in his first year of his nurse preparation programme, working with people living with learning disabilities. He had no experience of communicating with someone living with a learning disability. He was always fearful of triggering an outburst as he had heard from his peers of that happening sometimes.

Johann tried to think of things to say but found that people seemed to avoid him. When reflecting on this with his practice supervisor, Jenny, Johann identified that his body language was probably conveying his fear and making people avoid engaging with him. Johann and Jenny considered some strategies to overcome this.

- What strategies might you employ in a similar situation?
- Which of the 6Cs might this case study relate to?

There is an outline answer at the end of the chapter.

As this case study demonstrates, it is helpful to learn the art of asking questions. Nolan and Ellis (2008) describe several questioning techniques that nurses can employ. These include *open questions*, where patients are able to choose how to frame their answer, *closed questions*, where the answer is limited (often to yes or no), and *probing questions*, which seek more specific information. When communicating with people in the care setting, it is best to avoid the use of *multiple questions*, which are often used to query related problems. For example, asking about the nature of a particular symptom and what causes and relieves it in one sentence is likely to leave the patient confused as to which bit of the question to answer. Similarly, *leading questions*, which already contain the answer (e.g. 'You're in pain, aren't you?'), will elicit an answer from the patient affirming what has been said. Leading questions, as well as usually gaining an answer affirming what has been said, also cause the patient not to talk about what they want to talk about, thereby suppressing the patient's experience and not providing anything new.

Activity 3.4   Communication

When you are with your friends either socially or in the university, try asking these two different questions and consider the answers you get: 'How are you?' and 'Are you all right?'.

What do you notice about the responses you get? Why might this be? What does this mean for the sorts of questions you might ask in the workplace or patients?

There is an outline answer at the end of the chapter.

It needs to be remembered that when patients are in an unfamiliar setting, they may not be able to respond as quickly or as thoughtfully as usual and will often rely on the nurse's skills to help them relay the necessary information. Probing questions are useful for focusing on specific issues or gathering more detail on answers already given. Rhetorical questions, statements which do not require an answer, may be used as icebreakers. For example, commenting on the weather may be useful to start to relax the patient and build a dialogue. However, such statements also need to be used with caution in order not to make people feel they are being patronised. Other more useful ice-breakers could be used, such as introducing yourself, asking how the patient likes to be addressed, and checking whether they have any questions.

Different categories of question are useful for different stages of the assessment process because they serve different functions. Table 3.2 offers some examples.

Questioning may also identify areas that are outside your current scope of knowledge and require you to refer to others. Activity 3.5 will help you to identify the interplay of different forms of questioning.

Stage of nursing process	Type of question	Question content
Establishing baseline information	Closed questions	Can elicit biographical information such as name, date of birth, address, occupation, doctor, next of kin, whether a symptom is present or not, whether a procedure is consented to or not.
Problem identification	Open questions	Useful for gaining understanding of the reason for requiring health and social care intervention, symptomatic description, personal management of the problem.
Defining the problem	Probing questions	Can elicit what causes or alleviates the problem, clarification of patient explanation.

Table 3.2 Types of questioning used in the nursing process

Activity 3.5 Communication

Read the transcript below and identify where different forms of questions are being used.

Student: Good morning, Mrs Riley. My name is Chris and I am a student nurse. Welcome to the ward. I have a few questions that I need to ask you about your personal details and why you have come here today. Would that be all right?
Patient: Yes.
Student: Let's start with your details. What is your full name?
Patient: My full name is Patricia Anne Riley.
Student: And do you like to be called Patricia, Anne or Mrs Riley, or something shorter?
Patient: I prefer to be called Patricia.
Student: What is your address?
Patient: I live at 27 Long View Road, Brigstown, East Sussex.
Student: What is your telephone number?
Patient: 01443 56789.

Student: Who is your next of kin?

Patient: John Riley, my husband.

Student: Does he live at the same address and have the same telephone number?

Patient: He has a mobile number, which is 07798 45607.

Student: What has brought you here today?

Patient: I have been having these terrible pains when I go to the toilet and I have been passing rather a lot of blood recently.

Student: When you say going to the toilet, do you mean passing urine or having your bowels open?

Patient: I mean having my bowels open.

Student: Is there anything that you have noticed that makes the pain worse?

Patient: When I eat spicy foods.

Student: I presume you pass blood then as well? Have you been told what the problem might be?

Patient: The doctor said something about irritable bowel syndrome but also having to rule out other causes and needing to do some more tests.

Student: Did you understand what the doctor said?

Patient: Not really.

Student: Would you like me to get my practice supervisor to help explain what irritable bowel syndrome is and the tests that the doctor has ordered?

Patient: Yes please.

An outline answer is given at the end of the chapter.

When designing a set of questions, Brinkmann and Kvale (2014), when discussing research question schedules, suggest that they start from the least invasive questions about actions to the more invasive ones about beliefs and values. Moving from the general to the more specific, allows people to adjust to what is being asked and a rapport to be established. Making use of reflective prompt cues, also known as Kipling's six honest serving men (Kipling, nd), can also be helpful. For example:

- Why – 'Why were you seeing your GP?'
- What – 'What were you doing just before the pain started?'
- Where – 'Where did you feel the burning sensation?'
- When – 'When do you feel the pain sensation?'
- Who – 'Who helps you with your care?'
- How – 'How does this make you feel?'

Completing Activity 3.6 will help you to practise different questioning techniques in a safe environment as well as consider your style of communication.

Activity 3.6 Communication

This activity is designed to enable you to practise different questioning techniques in order to gain an understanding of why and how information might be withheld by people and explore what you might do about this.

1. Spend about fifteen minutes finding out as much as possible about the health of a peer or a family member. Be sure to reassure them about confidentiality and gain their consent by telling them what you are doing.
2. Now compare the questions you asked with those you might ask as a health professional.
3. Were there any differences, and why might this be?
4. What further information do you need?
5. Did you suspect that some information was being withheld?
6. What alerted you to this, and what did you do?

An outline answer is given at the end of the chapter.

Gathering information can be problematic for several reasons. Some of these are listed below:

- Knowing what you are looking for – patients present with many different problems and sometimes they do not even know where to start explaining a *symptom*.
- Understanding what the patient is trying to say – this is likely to be related to the reason why you are seeing the patient in the first place, but sometimes people with limited experience struggle to make sense of what is being said to them and do not know what probing questions to ask to gain the information they need. Some people also have a limited vocabulary and struggle to find the words to explain what they are experiencing while other people use language, and specifically some words, to mean different things.
- Accurate recording and documentation – if records are not kept accurately and recorded in a timely manner, important information may be missing or difficult to find.
- Patient memory and ability to articulate it – patients may not be able to remember key points or be able to explain them; this is where asking a carer or family member can help to get a picture of the problem.
- Technology – technological breakdown can mean that important information is not accessible.
- Institutional differences – ways of collecting, collating and storing information can vary between institutions, making it difficult to make sense of some of the information that healthcare professionals have gathered.
- Archiving – archives can sometimes be difficult to access.

Patients may also not always be truthful in the information they give for various reasons. For example, ambulatory care settings, where people require care for less than

24 hours, often require there to be a responsible adult at home with the patient following certain procedures or day surgery. A patient may not want to admit that there is no one because they want to go home. Equally, the patient may be afraid that the procedure will not go ahead. And yet if something goes wrong at home as a consequence, the communication, assessment and decision-making processes of the nurse will also be scrutinised. It is therefore important to reflect on your own problem-solving and identify what options are available to you. Identifying nursing priorities is the next step after talking to the patient. We move forward now to consider areas to focus upon when analysing patient information.

Identifying nursing priorities through analysis of patient information

Part of the nurse's role is to analyse the information received from the patient and by other means, such as from carers and patient notes, in order to identify what needs to be done. Carpenito-Moyet (2016) suggests three main areas of focus when analysing patient information for nursing priorities:

1. strengths – areas that the patient can draw upon to progress to a previous or new health state;

2. risk factors – those things that might hold the patient back from recovery or progression; and

3. problems in functioning – areas that are not working properly.

A case study is offered to illustrate these points.

Case study: Bella's loss of sense of self

Bella is 45 and has come into the neurological unit because of a multiple sclerosis (MS) relapse that has affected her mobility, sight, and bladder and bowel control. She has had MS for 15 years and is usually relatively self-caring. She has had six relapses in the last 15 years. The last two relapses have had a profound effect on her mobility each time, which is why she has been admitted to hospital. She is also due to receive a course of intravenous medication to try to deal with some of the effects of the relapse.

You are the nurse admitting Bella. You observe that she is using two sticks to walk, is very wobbly and uncoordinated, and appears to be taking time to absorb information and answer your questions. When you ask her to remove her cardigan so that you can record her blood pressure, she fumbles with the buttons. You start to think:

(Continued)

(Continued)

- What are the significant nursing features?
- What is the patient's nursing care priority?

You identify that Bella has had MS for 15 years, and therefore has built up her knowledge and coping strategies for dealing with the illness (strengths to draw on). You start by asking her what her immediate concerns are. She identifies that although her mobility has been badly affected, of greater concern to her is her loss of bladder and bowel control, which has altered her view of herself as a woman and a wife (problems with functioning). She feels that without that sense of identity, she cannot deal with her other losses (i.e. mobility and visual acuity). Previously, she has always been able to problem-solve and look forward with hope to recovery and a return to a degree of normality. This time she is not so sure and feels hopeless (risk factors).

Together you identify that the priority is to involve the continence nurse to seek options and solutions. You discuss how she might cultivate a positive outlook to aid her recovery. You also consider how to solve functional problems by identifying what help she desires with washing and dressing, where to place the furniture to avoid obstacles, and how she might involve her husband in helping. You suggest the input of the occupational therapist for further advice on how to maintain her independent living. Finally, you discuss the planned medical treatment and its potential side effects, and what she might want to do to aid her recovery further when she goes home.

- How might the 6Cs relate to this scenario?

There is an outline answer at the end of the chapter.

The aspects relating to coping mechanisms, functional problems and altered self-image, as demonstrated in the case study, can then form the basis of your analysis of nursing priorities. Completing Activity 3.7 will help you to think about the nursing priorities in relation to Bella's case study.

Activity 3.7   Communication

Read the case study above about Bella again. How would you configure the nursing priorities within the scenario for a nursing handover?

An outline answer is given at the end of the chapter.

Not all aspects will fall within your scope of practice or expertise, and therefore will require onward referral or notification to other health and social care professionals, such as the doctor, continence nurse or occupational therapist. It is important that nurses are able to reach agreement with the patient about what these priorities are as part of person-centred care, which does not treat patients as objects, but as people concerned with their health and well-being and as collaborators in care. Working in such a way has been described as being in a skilled relationship that is based on viewing people as being in a relationship with themselves, with those around them, the situation and the larger world (Dewing, 2004; McCormack, 2004).

As the case study demonstrates, working with the patient is important, but is also something that can become lost in the busy health or social care environment. And yet how can we understand how people feel, what their symptoms are, or expect them to engage with self-management, if they are not involved in discussing their own care and in subsequent decision-making? As the healthcare environment changes and more patients are cared for in the community in their own homes, supporting them in their self-management is increasingly important. Consequently, nursing priorities need to reflect and incorporate patient priorities in order to promote the continuity of care and recovery. Having identified these nursing priorities together, it is important to be able to ensure the patient understands what they mean and that they are able to make sense of this explanation when working with other health professionals. The following section considers how to make sense of patient information.

Making sense of information and interpreting this to others

Professionals need to focus on becoming what Egan (2014) calls 'translator-practitioners' (page 29). What this means is having a good understanding of the relevant research and evidence base, as well as the practical possibilities to be able to communicate accurately, and in terms they can understand, with patients and other health professionals. Interpretation here means being able to clarify terms that may be profession-specific, as well as give an explanation of how they apply. Questions that you might want to ask yourself as part of this process are:

- What is the patient's reason for admission, or the patient's explanation/ understanding for their current situation?
- What are the trends and significance within the objective information available?
- What is the important subjective information in this case, and what does it tell me?
- Is there further information I need?
- How do I develop a handover report?

Reading the case study below and then completing Activity 3.8 will help you to identify the key points that need to be considered and passed on within a given situation.

Case study: Robert's deteriorating health

Robert is a 65-year-old man who has advanced chronic kidney disease and related hypertension. His condition has slowly been deteriorating and he has recently become quite depressed. He has difficulty sleeping and feels quite weak. He is under the care of the specialist community matron team where you are currently on placement.

He tells you that his wife normally takes care of him, but due to financial pressures she has had to take a part-time job. He feels deprived of company. His blood pressure readings are significantly raised, and when you check the nursing notes you see that these have been steadily rising. You note that he has had a recent blood test but does not know the result. He has an appointment in the pre-dialysis clinic scheduled for next week.

Activity 3.8   Critical thinking

List the important points you have identified from your interactions with Robert.

How would you formulate a documentary entry for informing other professionals about his situation and progress?

An outline answer is given at the end of the chapter.

Making sense of information means making sure you have gathered what you need and you understand it all in the first place. For example, do you know what causes chronic kidney disease and the effects it can have on people? Have you checked with Robert what he understands and how he copes? Do you know the management processes involved? Unless you understand the results of your questions, you cannot explain these to the patient and to other health professionals, such as the clinic nurse who Robert is going to see. Having made sense of a patient's information, it is also important to identify the nursing priorities with the patient in order to start formulating a care plan.

Conclusion and reflection

Finding all the patient information needed can sometimes be a process of detection as you follow up different clues and leads. This involves communicating not only with the patient, but also with a variety of people, often across different disciplines.

Reflection will enable you to develop your practice by tracking changes in the way you think and act and make sense of your responses (Esterhuizen, 2022). Completing Activity 3.9 will help you to make sense of how you gather and interpret information.

Activity 3.9   Reflection

Consider a recent experience where you were involved in gathering and interpreting patient information and answer the following questions:

- How did you go about gathering and interpreting the information, and what problems did you encounter?
- How did you address any problems?
- What other ways could you have used?
- Would you do the same again, and why?

Having reflected on how you gather and interpret information, draw up an action plan of what you are taking forward. For further guidance on making use of reflection, you might like to refer to Esterhuizen (2023).

As this activity is based on your own experiences, there is a limited outline answer at the end of the chapter.

Chapter summary

The processes of gathering and interpreting information are important to ensure the accuracy of patient assessment and care planning. This chapter has highlighted some of the techniques involved in developing a process of questioning and of working with subjective and objective information. It has focused on how to represent information to others involved in the patient's care and how to identify nursing priorities with the patient through analysis of the information received. You have been offered the opportunity to complete a variety of activities in order to help you to develop your communication and critical thinking skills and to reflect on how and why you carry out patient assessment and alternatives that might work differently.

Activities: brief outline answers

Activity 3.1   Reflection (Page 42)

In the case study, the objective information gained meant James Ashton had a blood transfusion and was given lifestyle advice. The more personal, subjective information identified that James was drinking because he felt isolated following retirement; this information was used to seek extra help for him from the support group. Dealing with the issue that caused the drinking might prevent a later relapse, which the transfusion and advice alone would not.

Activity 3.2   Critical thinking (page 45)

Patient circumstances that might make this difficult are reduced mental capacity, level of consciousness, effects of drugs, language ability, effects of illness and trust. Other methods for gathering information that you might use are making use of your senses, intuition, and medical devices such as monitors. You might also expand your sources to include family, friends and carers, as appropriate.

Case study: Johann's questioning experience (page 46)

Some strategies that you might think about could be to approach people as persons and develop a conversation by finding out what their interests are and talking about those. Being yourself is important. You could talk about a few of your interests as well, if it seems appropriate. This case study relates to communication – one of the 6Cs.

Activity 3.4   Communication (page 47)

What you may notice is that when you ask, 'How are you?' people answer in a variety of ways, some short and some explaining that they are not OK. If you ask, 'Are you all right?', more people will just say, 'Yes'. This is because the first is an open question and the second a closed one which is also leading; that is asking, 'Are you all right?' invites a brief response and suggests you want to hear they are.

In the clinical setting, failing to enable patients to answer an open question may mean a symptom is missed and therefore the plan of care is inaccurate.

Activity 3.5   Communication (page 48)

Student: Good morning, Mrs Riley. My name is Chris and I am a student nurse. Welcome to the ward. I have a few questions that I need to ask you about your personal details and why you have come here today. *Would that be all right? (closed question)*

Patient: Yes.

Student: Let's start with your details. *What is your full name? (closed question)*

Patient: My full name is Patricia Anne Riley.

Student: *And do you like to be called Patricia, Anne or Mrs Riley, or something shorter? (closed question)*

Patient: I prefer to be called Patricia.

Student: *What is your address? (closed question)*

Patient: I live at 27 Long View Road, Brigstown, East Sussex.

Student: *What is your telephone number? (closed question)*

Patient: 01443 56789.

Student: *Who is your next of kin? (closed question)*

Patient: John Riley, my husband.

Student: *Does he live at the same address and have the same telephone number? (multiple questions)*

Patient: He has a mobile number, which is 07798 45607.

Student: *What has brought you here today? (open question)*

Patient: I have been having these terrible pains when I go to the toilet and I have been passing rather a lot of blood recently.

Student: *When you say going to the toilet, do you mean passing urine or having your bowels open? (probing question)*

Patient: I mean having my bowels open.

Student: *Is there anything that you have noticed that makes the pain worse? (probing question)*

Patient: When I eat spicy foods.

Student: *I presume you pass blood then as well? (leading question) Have you been told what the problem might be? (closed question)*

Patient: The doctor said something about irritable bowel syndrome but also having to rule out other causes and needing to do some more tests.

Student: *Did you understand what the doctor said? (closed question)*

Patient: Not really.

Student: *Would you like me to get my practice supervisor to help explain what irritable bowel syndrome is and the tests that the doctor has ordered? (closed question)*

Patient: Yes please.

Activity 3.6   Communication (page 50)

You are likely to have used a more conversational and less formal questioning style with a peer or family member because your relationship is already established. Health professionals use more formal questioning techniques. You are likely to have been alerted to the withholding of information by a change in non-verbal behaviour, such as breaking of eye contact, fidgeting and breaks in sentence structure. Reasons for withholding information might be lack of trust, anxiety and not understanding the question. You might have thought of using reassurance, being open and honest about why you needed the information and what it would be used for, and adjusting your position to one that was open. When operating in the non-professional world, people may also withhold information that you just don't need to know because it is embarrassing.

Case study: Bella's loss of sense of self (page 51)

This case study relates to a number of the 6Cs. These include commitment to Bella by finding out what her priorities are, as well as compassion through understanding her struggle, caring through identifying ways to help her with activities of daily living, and competence in how the assessment is completed. Of course, this is all made possible by good communication and having the courage to probe and identify answers.

Activity 3.7   Communication (page 52)

Bella is 45 years old and was admitted with an MS relapse. Some of the symptoms, such as loss of mobility and loss of bladder control, have been distressing for her. She has also been psychologically impacted by this abrupt change to her body image. I have assessed the nursing priorities to be helping Bella with maintaining a safe environment and to support her psychological adjustment to this new reality.

Activity 3.8 Critical thinking (page 54)

Robert is feeling depressed. The reasons might include a loss of self-esteem because his wife has to go to work in order to ease their financial burden. He appears to be missing her company. His blood pressure rise may be linked to these factors, making him feel more stressed, but you also need to find out what the blood test was for and the result. Your documentary entry could go something like this:

> *01.04.2022: Attended Mr Watson today. His blood pressure was raised at 228/125 mmHg. The trend for this has been steadily rising over the last two weeks. He appeared lethargic and in a low mood today. On talking to him, he seems to be missing his wife's company and feels isolated. He had blood taken on 29.03.2022: results are being sought. He has an appointment in the pre-dialysis clinic on 08.04.2022. He may need a medication review and referral to the counsellor.*

Activity 3.9 Reflection (page 55)

Action planning involves identifying what you have learned and relating this to what you intend to do in practice:

> *Action plan: I had problems gathering patient information because the patient did not understand the terminology I was using. I changed my approach by using simpler terms, but this meant that I needed to understand what I was saying, and I was not clear on some areas myself. Next time I will make sure that I understand what I am trying to explain before I meet with patients. I intend to keep reading about this particular topic area and discuss with my practice supervisor to ensure the accuracy of my understanding.*

Further reading

Ellis, P (2023) *Evidence-Based Practice in Nursing* (5th edn). London: SAGE.

This book clarifies what is meant by evidence-based practice and how you can find and apply it.

Esterhuizen, P (2023) *Reflective Practice in Nursing* (5th edn). London: SAGE.

A guide to the variety of ways in which you can reflect on your practice in order to develop and improve future practice.

Grant, A and Goodman, B (2018) *Communication and Interpersonal Skills in Nursing* (4th edn). London: SAGE.

A useful introduction to communication and interpersonal skills for nursing students.

Howatson-Jones, L and Ellis, P (eds) (2008) *Outpatient, Day Surgery and Ambulatory Care.* Chichester: Wiley-Blackwell.

This book outlines the nursing role and procedures in a variety of ambulatory and outpatient settings and will help to develop your knowledge of nursing contexts.

Hutchfield, K (2010) *Information Skills for Nursing Students.* Exeter: Learning Matters.

A clear description of where to source information and ways of doing this; this book will help you to be effective in your search for relevant information.

McCabe, C and Timmins, F (2013) *Communication Skills for Nursing Practice* (2nd edn). Basingstoke: Palgrave Macmillan.

This book outlines the variety of ways in which nurses and midwives communicate with patients, each other and the wider team. It offers suggestions for developing your communication skills.

Useful websites

www.gpnotebook.co.uk

This website is a reference source that patients and professionals can use.

www.patients.uptodate.com

This website offers information about various medical conditions.

Chapter 4　Assessment tools

Peter Ellis

Chapter aims

After reading this chapter, you will be able to:

- understand why and when to use an assessment tool;
- identify the knowledge and skills needed to use assessment and screening tools and list some potential problems;
- understand a range of assessment tools, such as the Malnutrition Universal Screening Tool (MUST), the Waterlow score and the National Early Warning Score (NEWS2); and
- identify how to utilise information gained from patient assessment to achieve a nursing diagnosis and a plan of care.

Introduction

Case study: Collaborative use of a falls risk assessment tool

Ian was in the second year of his nurse preparation programme and his placement was with the intermediate care team. He noticed that many different professions, such as occupational therapists, physiotherapists and nurses, worked alongside each other in this area. This was particularly evident when they were applying the falls risk assessment tool, with the nurses completing one side relating to the patient's presenting history, social background, biographical information and nursing observations, and the therapists completing mobility and independence assessment elements. The resultant document was then integrated with the medical assessment, enabling a multidisciplinary plan of care to be generated.

Ian noted in his reflective diary the advantages of collaborative practice enacted in this way, reducing repetition for the patient and subjective judgement based on their particular profession's take on the situation. The falls risk assessment tool also triggered certain actions that needed to be followed up. Ian thought this could be especially useful for less experienced professionals such as himself.

It is important for students to gain an understanding of the relevance of assessment and screening tools and how to apply and interpret them so as to be able to accurately assess patient needs. Screening tools offer an important and structured basis for planning care interventions. As the case study above highlights, they can be used collaboratively and also offer important trigger points to prompt the planning and delivery of care. The information collected by screening tools is also useful for compiling audit data to identify the effectiveness of care. It is important that you understand the purpose and usefulness of a variety of screening tools to aid your patient assessment and care planning. This chapter will clarify the purpose of assessment tools as well as identify some potential problems with their use. It will introduce the MUST, Waterlow and NEWS2 screening tools, and identify how the information they collate is used to make a nursing diagnosis. The activities offered throughout the chapter will help you to reflect on your own knowledge and skills as well as make use of some of the screening tools with a case study. You will be invited to apply some of the principles to your own practice experience.

The purpose of assessment tools

The purpose of assessment tools is to enable you to carry out an effective assessment which is as objective as possible. Not only that, but the tools ensure the process is structured (so nothing is missed) and that other professionals are also able to understand the data collected and how it might be put to use. Wilson et al. (2018) state that assessment tools can be categorised by what they do:

- health screening and diagnosis – identifying the problem and its severity (e.g. the Hospital Anxiety and Depression Scale) (Pritchard, 2011);
- descriptive – describing the problem but not necessarily directing action (e.g. the Barthel Activities of Daily Living Index) (Mahoney and Barthel, 1965); and
- predictive – identifying the potential for problems to develop (e.g. the Braden Scale for Predicting Pressure Sore Risk) (Anthony, 2010).

What assessment tools do is offer a way to measure the problem, or consider potential problems, in an objective fashion that can be consistently communicated to other professionals. The negative aspect of this is that the terminology and process may not always be comprehensible to patients, and therefore can exclude them from the process. Completing Activity 4.1 will help you to identify your knowledge about the range of assessment tools that are used in practice and their purpose.

Activity 4.1 Critical thinking

Make a list of the assessment tools that you have seen used in your placements. Now consider:

- What was their purpose?
- Were other professionals involved in their use, and if so how and why?
- Were there any problems with using the tool?
- How was the patient involved?

As this activity is based on your experience, there is no outline answer at the end of the chapter.

You might have included some of the more commonly used assessment tools in your list, such as pressure ulcer scoring systems, pain assessment scales and the mini-mental score. You might have identified specific problems with patient involvement, such as the use of jargon, patient anxiety, cognitive ability and memory, and perhaps the time it might take to involve them. It is also important to remember that assessment tools are only as good as the knowledge and expertise of the person using them. The National Institute for Health and Care Excellence (NICE) has developed a range of guidelines that underpin and inform many assessment tools (**www.nice.org.uk**). The next section explains in more detail the importance of knowledge and skills for using assessment tools.

Knowledge and skills needed to use assessment tools

An inaccurately used assessment tool can put patients at risk because you may over- or underestimate their risk of a particular problem or make inappropriate use of resources. It is important to ensure that you have the knowledge, skills and time to use the assessment tool and to continue to develop this with a diversity of patients so that you can improve your skills and competence. Key aspects that need to be considered before using assessment tools are:

- knowledge of the tool – the purpose of using the tool and how relevant and suitable it is to the patient's situation;
- knowledge and understanding of the patient's presenting problem and the reason for using the tool to assess this;
- communication – understanding how to gain information and explain what you are doing;
- obtaining data – understanding how to use the tool;
- recording data and information – understanding how to record the results accurately;
- evaluation of data and information – being able to analyse the results; and
- linking results to diagnosis and care planning – being able to think critically about the results and analyse what to do next.

Consider the following case study and then complete Activity 4.2 in order to apply these principles.

Case study: Assessing pressure area risk

Niamh was working in a community placement with the district nurses in the first year of her preparation programme. They had a patient, Gladys, who was bed-bound. Niamh's practice supervisor, Maggie, explained that they needed to assess Gladys's pressure area

(Continued)

(Continued)

risk and asked Niamh whether she knew how to do this. Niamh replied that she had used the pressure risk assessment tool in hospital but was not sure if it was different in a community setting. Maggie showed Niamh how the pressure risk assessment tool was used in the community and then told her to have a go at assessing Gladys's needs. They discussed the results, which showed that Gladys was at high risk and needed specialist equipment.

Activity 4.2   Critical thinking

Now you have read the case study, see if you can answer the questions below:

- What questions does Niamh need to address before using the tool?
- What should she communicate to Gladys?
- How should she record the results?
- What might she need to consider within her analysis of the results?

An outline answer is given at the end of the chapter.

When using an assessment tool, it is important to explain as fully as possible to the patient what the tool is and why it is being used, to ensure patient consent. This is one reason why you need to understand how the tool works and what you hope to achieve in using it, in order to give an accurate description. Therefore, you need to address the following aspects when preparing to use an assessment tool so that you can justify what you are doing with the patient and communicate this to other professionals who may also be involved in the patient's care. Your explanation should include:

- the aim and objective(s) of using the assessment tool;
- the benefits and limitations of the assessment tool;
- showing you have ensured that the information gathered is accurate;
- what you plan to do with the information gathered; and
- any actions that have been triggered from using the assessment tool (think about possible nursing interventions and also whether you need to involve other people).

Being clear about why you are using a particular tool and what you hope to achieve provides justification for your actions and the opportunity for you to reflect on what you have learned from this instance of using the tool. It also raises the question, in some settings and on some occasions, as to whether the assessment should take place at all. Reflecting on these questions helps to develop your knowledge and skills further. Completing Activity 4.3 can help you to think about what you have learned from using assessment tools.

Activity 4.3   Reflection

Think about an assessment tool you have used a number of times. Now consider the different situations you have used this tool in. What was similar and what was different? Were there any problems, and how did you solve them? What do you think you have learned? Have you ever used an assessment tool and found that no-one is going to use the results?

As this activity is based on your experience, there is no answer at the end of the chapter.

You might have considered your use of pain assessment tools. You might have identified how variable the results could be because of subjective scoring and interpretation and difficulty with determining action. You might have learned that you needed to integrate the information from the assessment tool with other information available to you so that you can make informed decisions about care planning.

Potential problems

A potential problem with using assessment tools is that you can become overly reliant on them, and therefore do not take sufficient note of the variety of evidence, of which they are only a part (Wilson et al., 2018). Over-reliance on an assessment tool may mean that you miss other issues going on with the patient, putting them at risk. Equally, assessment tools may not be culturally sensitive, and therefore may miss out important aspects (e.g. diet content or the different ways people respond to or express pain). Continuously relying on assessment tools may also be deskilling because you use your clinical assessment skills less (Wilson et al., 2018). In order to provide holistic care, it is important that you use your clinical observation skills and therapeutic communication to involve patients in your application of relevant assessment tools for their care. If you do not involve patients, how do you know what they are experiencing? Completing Activity 4.4 will help you to consider the relevance of clinical assessment skills for holistic assessment.

Activity 4.4   Reflection

List the clinical assessment skills that are important for developing holistic and person-centred care. How could you develop these further? How could you increase patient involvement and ensure you are integrating the 6Cs?

An outline answer is given at the end of the chapter.

Making sure that you continue to develop all your assessment skills will help you to avoid some of the potential problems identified above. We now proceed to consider some selected assessment tools and how to use them.

Malnutrition Universal Screening Tool (MUST)

The MUST is used to identify those who are malnourished or at risk of becoming malnourished (Shah et al., 2022). It assesses body mass index (BMI) through height and weight measurements, establishes the percentage of unintentional weight loss according to tables provided, and scores subjective criteria such as the effects of acute disease, adding all these together to identify the overall risk (Goodhand and Ewen, 2022). The tool and explanatory information can be viewed at the British Association for Parenteral and Enteral Nutrition website (**www.bapen.org.uk**). Holmes (2010) emphasises that the MUST should be used in conjunction with clinical assessment information so that a nutritional support plan can be commenced and evaluated over time. Nutritional health is important for the body's ability to fight infection and for growth and repair (Cook, Shepherd and Boore, 2021). NICE (2017) recommends that screening should be undertaken for all patients on admission to hospital, a care home, or on their first outpatient appointment and repeated in those cases where there is clinical concern (**www.nice.org.uk/CG32**). Such patients include those with:

- BMI <18.5 kg/m²;
- unintentional weight loss >10% within the last 3–6 months;
- a BMI of less than 20 kg/m² and unintentional weight loss greater than 5% within the last 3–6 months; decreased absorptive capacity; and
- increased nutritional requirement (e.g. burns or other large wounds such as abdominal surgery).

Case study: Simon's ulcerative colitis flare-up

Simon was 19 years old and due to start university. He had been diagnosed with ulcerative colitis in his early teens. As he prepared to go to university, his symptoms of diarrhoea, abdominal cramps and general malaise worsened, and he started to lose weight. On his way to meet a friend, he collapsed and was taken to hospital. Following investigations in accident and emergency, he was diagnosed with an acute exacerbation of ulcerative colitis and admitted to the gastrointestinal ward. The student nurse, Geena, who was admitting Simon completed the MUST and noted that his BMI was 19, but that his weight loss was less than 5 per cent over the last three months. This gave Simon a MUST score of 1, which meant he was at medium risk of malnutrition. Geena documented Simon's MUST score and relayed the result to her practice supervisor, Peter. Peter explained that as Simon was at medium risk of malnutrition, they would write that his nutritional intake was to be observed in the care plan, and that Simon was to be rescreened with the MUST in three days' time. Geena asked why they were not referring Simon to the dietitian now. Peter explained that, as Simon was deemed to be medium risk, the objective was to see what Simon ate and if there was anything interfering with his food intake in order to make a considered judgement. He explained that not everyone at risk needed full multidisciplinary team input immediately and that there is often a need to get more than one score for an individual in order to see if a pattern is emerging.

Over the next day, it was noted that cramping pain was interfering with Simon eating. His pain relief was adjusted, and as his medication to counteract the ulcerative colitis symptoms took effect, Simon began to eat more regularly. His repeat MUST screen indicated that Simon was now low risk and he was discharged home.

In Simon's case study, you will have noted that his absorptive capacity has been reduced by the flare-up of his ulcerative colitis, putting him at medium risk of malnutrition despite his age. Completing Activity 4.5 will help you to identify some other patient situations where using the MUST would be indicated.

Activity 4.5   Critical thinking

Consider what diseases and other signs and symptoms of disease might make you think a patient needed to be screened for malnutrition and make a list.

An outline answer is given at the end of the chapter.

In practice, you may find that you will be using a number of assessment tools concurrently, especially with very sick patients. What is also important is that you use assessment tools to help pick up issues that you might otherwise have missed. Only using an assessment tool once a problem is well established will not benefit the patient. It is also important, as we saw in Simon's case study, that you understand that assessment tools are useful for establishing a baseline and therefore may often need to be applied a number of times over a period of time. A good example of this is in the care home setting, where a person may lose weight over a prolonged period of time and this may be missed by staff unless they repeatedly weigh the individual and apply tools such as MUST on a regular basis.

The next tool we will consider is the Waterlow pressure ulcer risk assessment tool, which draws on some of the results from the MUST score.

Waterlow pressure ulcer risk assessment tool

The Waterlow pressure ulcer risk assessment tool was developed by Judy Waterlow in 1985. She recognised the economic and human cost of pressure ulcers, and has continued to revise and update the scoring system to include later research (Waterlow, 2008). The scoring system considers risk categories that are scored according to the patient's presentation. The scores are then added together to identify the overall risk. The categories include:

- BMI;
- visual assessment of skin type;
- age and sex (gender);
- malnutrition screening;
- continence;
- mobility; and
- special risks such as surgery, trauma, disease effects and neurological deficits.

The overall risk is defined as *at risk, high risk* or *very high risk*, and a range of pressure-reducing aids and nursing care options is proposed in order to manage the level of risk identified (Waterlow, 2008). The latest Waterlow scoring system can be viewed at **www.judy-waterlow.co.uk**, and you can download a useful quick guide. Completing Activity 4.6 will help you to identify the local version used in your practice area.

Activity 4.6 Critical thinking

Look at the quick guide on the Waterlow website (**www.judy-waterlow.co.uk**). Now consider the pressure scoring system you have seen used in your practice or look for one on your next placement. Are there any differences and, if so, what might be the reasons? What is the local policy for which assessment tool is used and how you should respond according to what it shows?

As this activity is based on your experience and practice area, there is no answer at the end of the chapter.

Local policy takes account of research, national guidelines and other relevant assessment tools such as those used for wound assessment. Local policy may also be influenced by the types of patients being cared for whose inherent risks for health issues, such as pressure ulcers, may differ from those of the general hospital population. It is important that you inform yourself of local policies and guidelines in order to be able to evaluate your use of assessment tools and their effectiveness. Local policies are developed through practitioner feedback as well as research and national guidelines and are an intrinsic element of the evidence-base for nursing practice (Ellis, 2023). We now proceed to consider the NEWS2 scoring system.

National Early Warning Score (NEWS2)

There have been a number of early warning systems used in the care of acutely ill patients. The multiplicity of such systems used in healthcare institutions led to the development of a national standard because of differences in local systems and language and the confusion this sometimes created. The NEWS score was developed to provide acute care teams with a system that enabled recognition of changes in the condition of, and a timely response to, acutely ill patients. NEWS was updated in 2017 to produce the NEWS2 scoring system.

Early detection and a competent, timely clinical response are the key determinants of the outcome for people who are acutely ill and can even prevent the need for intensive care (Vincent et al., 2018). The NEWS assessment tool was developed as a standardised scoring system to warn of physiological changes in the condition of patients who were very unwell, so that timely interventions could be implemented (Royal College of Physicians, 2012). NICE (2007) had previously recommended that acutely ill patients needed to be monitored more closely to identify deterioration in the acute hospital setting (**www.nice.org.uk/CG50**). The NEWS2 assessment tool integrates six simple fields to measure physiological parameters, forming the basis of the scoring system. These are:

1. respiration rate;

2. oxygen saturation;

3. systolic blood pressure;

4. pulse rate;

5. level of consciousness or new confusion; and

6. temperature.

The specialised observation chart uses colours to denote when observation results are entering danger trigger zones. You will see these used in acute settings such as surgical and medical wards, as well as intensive care and accident and emergency. When you next have an acute placement, examine the observation charts used and ask practitioners how they use them. Notably, NEWS2, when used with patients presenting with COVID-19, has been shown to underestimate risk, with recommendations being made that any new version of the tool might include more focus on respiratory compromise (Bradley et al., 2020).

There are many other assessment tools available, such as falls, pain, anxiety, informational needs, self-esteem and body image, sedation scores, and wound assessment, and different variations are also sometimes used according to the diseases or conditions the patient has presented with (see recommended reading for more sources of assessment tools). We have focused on just three of the most widely used assessment tools here. These are all applicable to the following case study.

Case study: Mr Jordan's biliary stent

Mr Jordan is a 70-year-old man who has liver cancer. He has become more jaundiced and unwell. Although his condition is terminal, there are palliative procedures that can help him. One of these is a biliary stent insertion, which will help relieve pressure in the biliary duct and reduce the jaundice by allowing the bile to drain into the small bowel again, for a while. Mr Jordan has lost a considerable amount of weight in the last month as he has lost his appetite and has felt quite nauseous. On admission, his BMI is less than 18.5 and his skin is noted to be dry and warm. His vital signs are temperature 37.8°C, pulse 100 bpm, respirations 15 breaths/minute, blood pressure 130/85 mmHg. His urine output is 70 ml/hour. The biliary stent procedure is undertaken in the radiology department, requiring Mr Jordan to lie on a hard X-ray table for up to three hours. As it is a painful procedure, Mr Jordan is given pre-emptive analgesia of morphine and the sedative midazolam. The procedure is carried out successfully and Mr Jordan returns to the ward after three hours. The next day, his temperature starts to rise, and over the next few days his condition deteriorates. His vital signs are now temperature 40.1°C, pulse 50 bpm, respirations 24 breaths/minute, blood pressure 200/110 mmHg. His urine output has fallen to 20 ml/hour. Mr Jordan is now also delirious. Blood cultures confirm that Mr Jordan has septicaemia. He is moved to a high-dependency unit for further monitoring. Intravenous antibiotics are started, and Mr Jordan gradually improves. After a week, he is well enough to move out of the high-dependency unit. However, it is noted that he has developed a sacral pressure sore.

Read the above case study again and then use the assessment tools (Waterlow, MUST and NEWS2) discussed earlier to complete Activity 4.7.

Activity 4.7   Critical thinking

After reading the case study, use each of the Waterlow, MUST and NEWS2 assessment tools in turn and try to complete the tool you have chosen using the information provided. Now consider the following questions:

- What are the benefits and limitations of this tool in relation to Mr Jordan?
- What are the issues of using this tool with Mr Jordan (e.g. do you have all the information you need or is some missing, and, if so, how will you find it)?
- What skills do you need?
- What actions are triggered by the use of the tool with Mr Jordan?
- Who else might you need to involve?

An outline answer is given at the end of the chapter.

As you will have noted, the assessment tools all come to different conclusions. You need to analyse these conclusions and identify your nursing diagnosis of the situation. This is considered further in the next section.

Relationship of screening tools to making a nursing diagnosis

Screening tools help to identify the problems the patient has. The information provided by the assessment tool is analysed by practitioners to determine what to do next. Part of this analysis process is making a nursing diagnosis based on the results obtained, to direct further action and nursing interventions. Making a nursing diagnosis is what practitioners do when they are interacting with patients (e.g. identifying whether a patient is anxious or in pain). It is important to be able to communicate what the nursing diagnosis is to the patient and to other professionals so that they can understand why you are following a particular course of action. The following case study illustrates how this is done.

Case study: Making a nursing diagnosis of infection

Erica was a 58-year-old woman who was having her leg ulcers redressed by the community nurse, Alicia. Alicia used a wound assessment chart to assess the progress of Erica's leg ulcers. Wound assessment charts vary between organisations, but commonly consider the dimensions of the wound, the appearance of the wound bed and surrounding skin, any exudate or bleeding, the level of pain, and the location of the wound to be entered on the body diagram (Dougherty et al., 2015). An example of a wound assessment chart can be found at the following link: **www.health careimprovementscotland.org/our_work/patient_ safety/tissue_viability_resources/general_wound_assessment_chart.aspx**.

When completing the assessment, Alicia noted that Erica was experiencing increasing discomfort. She examined Erica's leg ulcers and noted an increase in exudate and that the wound bed was showing signs of infection. Alicia made a nursing diagnosis of wound infection and altered the dressing regime. She explained to Erica why she was doing this. She also documented the change and her reasoning for this and communicated the change to Erica's GP.

The case study highlights how nurses make decisions about nursing interventions. These are based on the information gleaned from patients in a variety of ways. Being able to make a nursing diagnosis is important because you need to justify any changes you make to a patient's care. We will look at how to make a nursing diagnosis in greater detail in Chapter 5. Next, we consider how screening tools contribute to audit.

Screening tools and audit

Screening tools are used within the audit process because they provide consistent and more objective assessment of a phenomenon. For example, pressure sore prevalence audits are recommended to be undertaken regularly to benchmark, and improve, the quality of patient care (Clark et al., 2017). Audit collects and measures available information with the purpose of measuring care against evidence-based benchmarks (Barker, 2013). The European Pressure Ulcer Advisory Panel classification system differentiates between other wounds and pressure sores, helping practitioners to make this distinction in a systematic way (Clark et al., 2017). Completing Activity 4.8 will help you to identify the link between other assessment tools and audit.

Activity 4.8   Critical thinking

Make a list of any clinical audits you have seen completed in practice, or if you have not seen any, ask your practice supervisor which audits are carried out in your placement area. What information is collected and what tools are used to collect it? How do the results inform practice?

An outline answer is given at the end of the chapter.

You might like to explore the relevance of audit further by reading Ellis's (2023) *Evidence-Based Practice in Nursing*. Accurate assessment and interpretation of information obtained from audits are important to inform evidence-based nursing practice and promote high-quality patient care.

Conclusion

Assessment tools are useful for gaining information about problems, or potential problems, that patients may experience, as well as playing an important part in auditing the quality of care. They use a systematic approach and provide suggested further action, which is especially helpful to less experienced practitioners. Nevertheless, they should not take the place of other forms of clinical assessment such as observing and talking to patients to identify what they need.

Chapter summary

This chapter has examined the importance and relevance of assessment tools to patient assessment. The benefits and limitations of using assessment tools have been considered. Three of the most commonly used assessment tools – MUST, Waterlow and NEWS2 – have been referred to. It is important to recognise that the assessment tool is only as effective as the knowledge and skill of the person using it. Therefore, a range of activities to develop your knowledge and skills have been integrated into the chapter. Reflection on their use will help you to become more effective and accurate in your patient assessments and in making a nursing diagnosis.

Activities: brief outline answers

Activity 4.2   Critical thinking (page 64)

Niamh needs to find out what is wrong with Gladys in order to determine the suitability of the assessment tool and how to interpret the results. She will also need to check with her practice supervisor whether her understanding of the tool, gained from using it in the hospital setting, is appropriate for the community setting before starting to use it with Gladys. Niamh will need to explain to Gladys what she intends to do and why, and gain her consent. She will then need to use the assessment tool prompts to gather the data, record the results on the tool paperwork and then interpret the results, again explaining these to Gladys and explaining what the next actions are. She will need to record these in the nursing notes. Lastly, she will need to evaluate her use of the tool reflectively with her practice supervisor in order to inform her future practice.

Activity 4.4   Reflection (page 65)

Clinical assessment skills include questioning techniques and attentive listening (to review these, return to Chapter 3), observation and analytical thinking. Analytical thinking in particular aims to integrate all the assessments undertaken by a variety of professionals so that appropriate interventions can be commenced. You could develop your clinical assessment skills further by practising them regularly with each patient you encounter and making sure you are always taking a complete view of the patient's care needs rather than concentrating on one issue. You could involve patients more by asking them about their experience and offering information and explanation. You can integrate the 6Cs through developing your competence and through communicating appropriately to find out the patient's perspective. In this way, you can also demonstrate your commitment to care.

Activity 4.5   Critical thinking (page 67)

Problems that could result in a BMI of <18.5 include eating disorders such as anorexia nervosa and bulimia, mental illness such as depression, and physical illnesses such as cancer, particularly when patients are having chemo- or radiotherapy and when they are in the palliative stages. Sudden unexplained weight loss is often a sign of cancer. In the elderly, it may be because they do not have an appetite, for a variety of reasons, or have swallowing difficulties. Decreased absorptive capacity problems include Crohn's disease and ulcerative colitis and certain types of bowel surgery. Increased nutritional requirements are exerted by large wounds such as extensive pressure ulcers and burns and also by prolonged infection. Aspects that might alert you could include:

- mood and mental state;
- picking at food;
- lack of interest in appearance or hygiene;
- withdrawal from communication;
- vomiting and diarrhoea; and
- pain.

Activity 4.7   Critical thinking (page 70)

Using the MUST on Mr Jordan, you will have identified that he is at high risk of malnutrition. You do not know the percentage of weight he has lost but take into account his subjective view that it is considerable. The benefits of using the MUST is that it identifies Mr Jordan's nutritional risk, but its limitation is that it is based on a cognitively aware patient. The skills you need for using the tool are knowledge of how to use it and professional judgement of the patient problem and its likely health effects. The action triggered by the MUST is nutritional support. You would involve the dietitian to advise.

Using the Waterlow score in Mr Jordan's case, you will have identified that he is at high risk to very high risk of developing a pressure sore. You do not know the effect of lying on a hard X-ray table or how much weight he has lost. You consider the benefit of using this scoring system as identifying Mr Jordan's pressure risk but note its limitations in that it is based on your subjective interpretation as well as having a tendency to overestimate. The skills you need to use the tool are observational and analytical. The main issues of using this tool in this patient's case are his changing condition and needs. The actions triggered are to provide pressure-relieving aids, ensure appropriate manual handling techniques are used, and grade the pressure sore and apply dressing in accordance with local policy. For this, you might involve the local tissue viability nurse.

Using the NEWS2 assessment tool, you would have identified that Mr Jordan's vital signs and level of consciousness have triggered the need for more frequent recording of observations and for review of Mr Jordan by the intensive care outreach team. You consider the benefits of using this assessment tool as alerting you to Mr Jordan's deterioration and of involving other relevant professionals at an early stage. You may consider one of the limitations of the tool is that some patients may score on the cusp of, or just inside, a danger trigger zone, and this can lead to uncertainty of what to do. The skills needed to use this tool are being able to carry out accurate nursing observations and understanding the significance of these observations. The actions triggered are more frequent nursing observations and involvement of the outreach team, as well as notifying the radiology team who carried out the biliary stenting procedure.

Activity 4.8   Critical thinking (page 72)

The type of audits carried out in practice are likely to include mortality rates following medical intervention, resuscitation outcomes, pressure ulcer incidence, infection rates and record-keeping. What these have in common is that an assessment tool for finding out the information will be used. Assessment is therefore also important for practice in order to continue practice development. In care settings you might also see audits, including for medication use, care plan quality and infection control, widely used.

Further reading

Ellis, P (2023) *Evidence-Based Practice in Nursing* (5th edn). London: SAGE.

This book has a clear section on the importance of audit and will help to inform your thinking about this.

Wilson, B, Woollands, A and Barrett, D (2018) *Care Planning: A Guide for Nurses* (3rd edn). Harlow: Pearson Education.

This book has a useful section on the advantages and disadvantages of assessment tools and will help you to set their use within the wider context of care planning.

Useful websites

www.bapen.org.uk

This website gives information about the MUST score.

www.judy-waterlow.co.uk

This website identifies how to use the Waterlow scoring system.

www.nice.org.uk

This website offers information on NICE guidelines.

www.nice.org.uk/CG32

This link takes you to the page for Clinical Guideline 32, which offers specific information on nutritional assessment.

www.nice.org.uk/CG50

This link takes you to the page for Clinical Guideline 50, which gives specific information on the assessment of deterioration in acutely ill adults.

https://nursingnotes.co.uk/resources/guide-nursing-assessments/

A really useful list of assessment tools nurses and others might use.

https://www.rcplondon.ac.uk/projects/outputs/national-early-warning-score-news-2

This is the Royal College of Physicians page which is dedicated to the tools used in NEWS 2 as well as their interpretation.

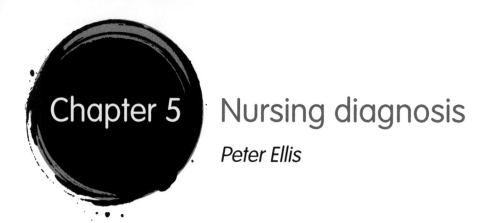

Chapter 5 Nursing diagnosis

Peter Ellis

NMC Future Nurse: Standards of Proficiency for Registered Nurses

This chapter will address the following platforms and proficiencies:

Platform 3: Assessing needs and planning care

At the point of registration, the registered nurse will be able to:

3.1 demonstrate and apply knowledge of human development from conception to death when undertaking full and accurate person-centred nursing assessments and developing appropriate care plans.

3.2 demonstrate and apply knowledge of body systems and homeostasis, human anatomy and physiology, biology, genomics, pharmacology and social and behavioural sciences when undertaking full and accurate person-centred nursing assessments and developing appropriate care plans.

3.3 demonstrate and apply knowledge of all commonly encountered mental, physical, behavioural and cognitive health conditions, medication usage and treatments when undertaking full and accurate assessments of nursing care needs and when developing, prioritising and reviewing person-centred care plans.

3.5 demonstrate the ability to accurately process all information gathered during the assessment process to identify needs for individualised nursing care and develop person-centred evidence-based plans for nursing interventions with agreed goals.

3.15 demonstrate the ability to work in partnership with people, families and carers to continuously monitor, evaluate and reassess the effectiveness of all agreed nursing care plans and care, sharing decision making and readjusting agreed goals, documenting progress and decisions made.

3.16 demonstrate knowledge of when and how to refer people safely to other professionals or services for clinical intervention or support.

Platform 5: Leading and managing nursing care and working in teams

At the point of registration, the registered nurse will be able to:

5.4   demonstrate an understanding of the roles, responsibilities and scope of practice of all members of the nursing and interdisciplinary team and how to make best use of the contributions of others involved in providing care.

Chapter aims

After reading this chapter, you will be able to:

- define what is meant by a nursing diagnosis;
- explain the history and development of a nursing diagnosis;
- identify how a nursing diagnosis relates to the nursing process;
- consider some of the potential pros and cons of a nursing diagnosis for the patient and nurse; and
- develop a nursing diagnosis using the patient assessment.

Introduction

Creating a nursing diagnosis is the process by which nurses establish nursing priorities following their communication and interaction with patients. This chapter explains what a nursing diagnosis is and how you can develop one. It identifies some of the advantages and disadvantages of a nursing diagnosis and what this means for both the patient and the nurse.

What is meant by nursing diagnosis?

Wilkinson (2016) defines a nursing diagnosis as:

A concise label that describes patient conditions observed in practice. These conditions may be actual or potential problems or wellness diagnoses.

(page 6)

The important point here is that a nursing diagnosis requires accurate description of the main characteristics of the conditions observed. However, this presents problems because the ways terminology is used may vary between different professions and professionals, and therefore standardisation of terms helps to ensure consistency (Carpenito-Moyet, 2016). For example, a doctor might talk about hypoglycaemia whereas a nurse may describe this as low blood sugar. Nurses and other healthcare professionals increasingly try to demystify medical terminology to help patients to understand what they have been told, but what Carpenito-Moyet (2016) is suggesting is that nurses also need to be consistent in the terminology they use. The following case study identifies how a nursing diagnosis is established.

Case study: Su's informational needs

Su is a 53-year-old woman who has recently had her first breast screening appointment. She is recalled to the clinic for further imaging due to an abnormality being found. Su is very nervous and concerned. She has further radiological images taken, followed by a breast biopsy, and sees the breast physician for the results a week later. Su is told that she has a fibroadenoma – a benign tumour. As it is small, nothing further needs to be done. Su goes home relieved. However, when talking it over with her husband, Su starts to worry. The word 'tumour' sticks in her mind. Su equates the word 'tumour' with cancer. Su begins to find it difficult to sleep and eat and is anxious most of the time. She is worried that the benign tumour may develop into a cancerous one. She goes to see the nurse at her GP surgery. Hayley, the nurse, makes a nursing diagnosis of informational need. Hayley explains to Su that a fibroadenoma is a small knot of fibrous and glandular cells. These cells are a normal component of breast tissue but have multiplied too much. The breast biopsy has confirmed the medical diagnosis, that the cells are benign. 'Benign' means that the cells will not become cancerous and spread, but stay in their present location. Removal of the lump is only indicated if the fibroadenoma is particularly large. Hayley advises Su to become familiar with the feel of the lump so she can notice and act on any changes. In this way, Su can regain some control. After seeing Hayley, Su feels much better. She remembers that the breast physician did explain some of this to her, but she was too agitated at the time to take it in. Su also asks her husband to become familiar with the feel and shape of her breast and help to alert her to any change he may notice.

The case study above illustrates how the medical diagnosis of a benign fibroadenoma has left Su with further informational needs. This is partly because Su was too anxious to take in what was being said by the doctor, but also because she did not understand the medical jargon that the breast physician used. Hayley has listened to Su's concerns and from this has established a nursing diagnosis of *unmet need for information*. The case study shows that although medical and nursing diagnoses may be related, they often have differing foci and emphasis. The focus of the medical diagnosis is physiological; the focus of the nursing diagnosis in this case is on understanding the psychosocial impact of the physiological problem. Carpenito-Moyet (2016) asserts that nurses need to establish a classification system that describes not only the patient problem, but also patient responses, which are considered when making a nursing diagnosis. The key aspects of a nursing diagnosis are:

- defining the nursing problem (e.g. the person is unable to get out of bed);
- describing the characteristics of that problem using information from the patient and from objective assessment such as the use of an assessment tool (e.g. the patient says she cannot stand without support; a recent falls assessment identifies that she cannot balance due to right-sided leg weakness following a cerebrovascular accident);
- considering other relevant factors (e.g. level of visual acuity);
- considering different diagnoses for best fit (e.g. pain or arthritis causing immobility); and
- identifying what you hope to achieve (e.g. for the patient to be able to get out of bed as independently as possible).

(Wilkinson, 2016)

Nevertheless, trying to standardise terms should not distract nurses from clarifying information given to patients. Nursing diagnosis and medical diagnosis are different because the nursing emphasis is on a holistic assessment of the patient, which considers psychological as well as physical concerns (Wilson et al., 2018).

What a nursing diagnosis is not is simply stating a patient problem, such as 'cannot mobilise'. The problem needs to be defined. This means in reality that the nursing diagnosis needs to be clear about what 'cannot mobilise' actually means. It could mean:

- Cannot stand at all.
- Can stand in a stand aid to be transferred.
- Can mobilise with a frame.
- Can mobilise only with the support of carer(s).

In contrast, a medical diagnosis will focus on a health deficit, such as immobility, for example, which is established by the medical practitioner. Nursing diagnoses try to involve and include patients by taking account of their experience and how this feels for them. Completing Activity 5.1 will help you to reflect on your understanding of a nursing diagnosis.

Activity 5.1 Reflection

Think about your last placement and the patients you cared for. When you were new to the area, were you able to use the care plan, containing the nursing diagnosis in order to help you provide the care that patients there needed? Was the description of the conditions the patients had clear enough for them to be involved in planning how they could be enabled and empowered, and what the role of the nurse is in caring for them?

As this activity is based on your experience, there is a limited answer at the end of the chapter.

You may have identified that you carry out the instructions of others without always knowing how they are framing the nursing diagnosis or indeed that the verbal instructions are not reflected in the detail of the written nursing diagnosis. You may have thought about some of the descriptors used for patient problems, such as immobile, incontinent and unable to self-care. However, these are rather vague and could be more precise in order to help practitioners think about what to do, and perhaps more importantly the level of care the person has described themselves as needing.

Vague care plans have a number of potential pitfalls associated with them. These include:

- the provision of inconsistent care;
- the provision of unsafe care;
- causing frustration and irritation.

Dougherty et al. (2015) make the point that patient problems and nursing diagnoses may not always be phrased the same because other disciplines may not always see the problem in the same way. This is why it is important for nurses to take a holistic and multidisciplinary view in order to develop a nursing diagnosis that takes into account the involvement of other disciplines as well as the patient. In the next section, we consider how and why nursing diagnoses started to be used.

The history and development of nursing diagnosis

The history of nursing diagnosis grew out of the frustration of nurses with a biomedical view of illness and caring that focused on the disease and not the person, and which ignored nurses' observations of patient responses. Nursing diagnosis is not a new concept. Florence Nightingale was commenting over 160 years ago on the need for hospitals to keep records that enabled comparisons to be made on the effectiveness of care (Nightingale, 1859, cited in Weir-Hughes, 2007, page 35). Systematic methods of planning and evaluating patient care were introduced globally into nursing programmes of learning and practice in the 1970s (Gordon, 1994). In the US, nursing diagnoses began to be used in the 1950s and were gradually amalgamated into nursing practice through the efforts of the American Nurses Association and then later through the addition of further definition by the North American Nursing Diagnosis Association (NANDA) as part of the nursing process (Carpenito-Moyet, 2016). There will be further discussion of the nursing process in a later section.

Around the same time, Carper (1978) was developing her theories of nursing knowledge as being different from medical knowledge, and these have also informed the process of developing a nursing diagnosis. These theories see patients as unique, which they are, and with their own resources and strengths that need to be considered.

NANDA has defined and characterised many of the nursing diagnoses that patients are likely to present with in a variety of settings (see **www.nanda.org**). Examples include anxiety, grieving, hopelessness, acute pain, risk for violence, impaired mobility, deficient fluid volume, nutrition imbalance and many more (Carpenito-Moyet, 2016). Nurses are becoming more empowered through defining what the nursing diagnosis is, and this in turn is helping them to be clear in their definition of what nursing is. Completing Activity 5.2 will help you to understand this point.

Activity 5.2   Reflection

Think about when you first considered nursing as a career. What did you think nursing was all about and what it might involve? What informed your definition? What do you think nursing is now? What has changed?

An outline answer is given at the end of the chapter.

What you may have realised is that the nursing diagnosis is about identifying elements, or activities, within the life of the patient with which they need support at any given time. It is these individual issues, as defined by the patient in collaboration with the nurse, that nursing care focuses on rather than the more reductionist medical diagnosis. So, for example, the nursing diagnosis may see a person as needing support with pain relief, protection from pressure sore development, and help with washing, dressing and feeding (among other things), while the medical diagnosis may simply be 'fractured neck of femur'.

In essence, this nursing diagnosis is more about what individual patients experience and what they might experience rather than some more objective label. We move on now to consider some of the advantages and disadvantages of using nursing diagnoses.

Advantages and disadvantages of nursing diagnoses

No nursing process should be undertaken without first reflecting upon whether it is fit for purpose and likely to achieve what you are aiming for. There will be more on the nursing process in the next section. While it is acknowledged that discipline expertise between nursing and medicine overlaps in areas of disease prevention, taking a history, diagnosing medical problems and seeking consultant advice, there are also many areas of difference, particularly in relation to nursing and medical definition and management of problems (Carpenito-Moyet, 2016). Like most processes, nursing diagnoses come with advantages and disadvantages.

Advantages of nursing diagnoses:

- They clearly define the problem – it is important to be able to communicate patient problems clearly to nurses and other healthcare practitioners.
- They focus on the individual patient rather than all patients with similar conditions – patients are unique and nursing diagnoses reflect this.
- They consider nursing priorities, which may differ from medical ones – they consider problems from other scientific viewpoints such as the social sciences.
- They direct specific nursing action and evaluation of that action – nursing diagnoses provide the basis on which care is planned and evaluated.

(Hinchliff et al., 2008)

Therefore, by clearly defining the problem and the actions that should follow, information is passed between care providers regarding what the patient's needs are and criteria are established by which to measure outcomes. This may be particularly beneficial for novice nurses and those new to practice. It is also helpful in busy settings where there may be limited time for verbal handovers as well as in settings where the workforce may be transitory (for example, where a lot of agency staff are employed). Clear nursing diagnoses and subsequent plans of care enable nurses taking over the care of a patient to understand what is happening and provide some continuity of care. However, there are also some disadvantages, and potential disadvantages, of nursing diagnoses.

Disadvantages of nursing diagnoses:

- The patient does not understand the nursing diagnosis – patients need to be included in discussion when the nursing diagnosis is being drawn up so that they can see how the nursing diagnosis is different from the medical diagnosis.
- The terminology may not be easily transferable to different healthcare systems.
- Nursing diagnosis-directed interventions can be prescriptive – the actions asked for dictate what should be done and may not allow other interpretations according to unique patient circumstance.
- Nursing judgements can become formulaic, restricting learning.
- Care is fragmented – nursing diagnoses give specific directions to nursing interventions, which can deconstruct the act of nursing care to a task.

(Carpenito-Moyet, 2016)

Some of these disadvantages are avoidable when nurses are self-aware and do not try to impose their own values and understanding of the patient situation or make judgements about the patient. Imposition of values and judgements might be obvious where nurses start to refer to the patient according to the diagnosis rather than by name. Nurses also need to consider how the elements of the care that could fragment into tasks are driven by the patient's needs at any particular point in time and are delivered in a manner that is enabling and empowering. We now proceed to consider how nursing diagnosis relates to the patient assessment process.

How nursing diagnosis relates to the nursing process

The nursing process is a systematic way of problem-solving that includes the stages of assessing, planning, implementing and evaluating care. It includes critically thinking about potential nursing interventions to develop a care plan and then evaluating the outcomes of the care provided. The nursing process has been used for some time in the UK because it can help to articulate evidence-based nursing care (Dyson, 2004). Establishing the nursing diagnosis is a key part of the nursing process because it identifies what the nursing priorities are. The nursing process is cyclical and begins with patient assessment, which – combined with communication with the patient – helps the nurse to develop the nursing diagnosis. This is an important leadership role for nurses as they take the lead in developing a nursing diagnosis in order to plan nursing care for their patient(s).

Nurses use information obtained through patient assessment to make clinical judgements about the nursing care the patient needs. These clinical judgements are the nursing diagnoses (Dougherty et al., 2015). This suggests that there is a definite process to making a nursing diagnosis and subsequent decisions about care. Carpenito-Moyet (2016) identifies that patients are the starting point in the experiences and symptoms they describe, the signs they display, and their responses to medical and other health and social care interventions. Wilson et al. (2018) state that using a systematic process to develop a nursing diagnosis enables problems to be identified and solutions found. These are important considerations when trying to identify possible nursing problems, and from this a possible nursing diagnosis is made. Figure 5.1 shows the stages in the nursing process with the addition of the nursing diagnosis between assessment and planning, as suggested by Wilson et al. (2018).

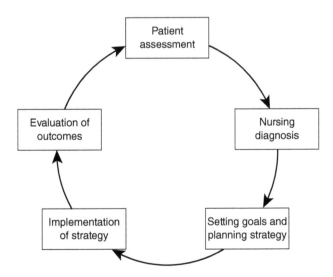

Figure 5.1   Nursing diagnosis as part of the nursing process

We have already established that because a systematic nursing diagnosis focuses not only on disease processes or treatment options, but also on nursing priorities, the outcomes looked for by nurses may be different from those sought by medical practitioners; although there are some nurse theorists who identify how this distinction is becoming eroded as nurses take on advanced nurse practitioner roles and adopt medical models of care (McCarthy and Jones, 2019). What is also important to recognise at this point is that nursing diagnoses and nurses' use of them also varies widely between nurses (D'Agostino et al., 2018). That said, accurate documentation of the nursing diagnosis process and implementation of the nursing actions planned are important for continuing effective and safe patient care (Ackley et al., 2022). The following case study illustrates how nursing diagnosis fits into the nursing process of assessment and care planning.

Case study: Diagnosing Bill's inability to cope

Bill is a retired postman. He is married with two grown-up children, one of whom lives in New Zealand and the other has a high-powered job in London. Bill's wife died six months ago and he has lost interest in looking after himself. His GP has become concerned that Bill is depressed and has referred him to the community adult mental health team. Gillian, the mental health nurse, visits Bill at home. She notices the dirty state of the house and unwashed cups and dishes in the kitchen. She also sees the stubble on Bill's chin and smells body odour. She asks Bill how he has been getting on and how things are since his wife died. Bill looks sad and starts to cry. Gillian remains silent but places a hand on Bill's to offer comfort. Gillian gives Bill time by moving on to discuss his current medication regime prescribed by his GP. When Bill is more composed, Gillian asks how he has been managing to look after himself. Bill says he has no appetite and sits most days in front of the television for company. Gillian asks him whether he has had any bereavement counselling.

Gillian makes a nursing diagnosis of inability to cope, which she defines as Bill not being able to carry out normal activities and avoiding people. She plans with Bill what to do. She finds out that Bill belongs to a local church, although he has not been since his wife died. Gillian gains Bill's agreement for her to talk to the vicar to come and see him and organise some help with cooking and cleaning from the congregation. Gillian also arranges for a Cruse group member to come and speak to Bill. When Gillian visits Bill the following week, he appears a bit more alert and interested. The visit of the Cruse group member has had a profound impact on him. He is talking about going to a group support session. Gillian sees this as regaining some ability to cope.

The above case study illustrates how nurses can define nursing problems, in this case a psychosocial issue, and find solutions by working with patients. Gillian was clear about the problem but did not try to impose solutions based on her own values; she worked with the activities and people already known to Bill. Nevertheless, involving others can sometimes also create problems when those people are not party to the initial diagnosis meeting, but are called upon to contribute in some way to the delivery of care. Therefore, continuous evaluation of the implementation phase of the nursing process is important to check on its validity and effectiveness for patient care.

Potential benefits and problems of nursing diagnosis for the patient and nurse

One of the benefits of accurate nursing diagnosis is that it can help promote effective patient care, and thereby potentially reduce the length of time that care is required (Weir-Hughes, 2007). What this means is that patients are able to return to their normal routines and leave care settings earlier because nurses focus on different outcomes to medicine (Welton and Halloran, 2005). Notably, nursing diagnoses are also, at least in some circumstances, predictive of not only the amount of care a patient will need, but also how long they may need it for (D'Agostino et al., 2017). In this way, nurses are able to demonstrate systematically the contribution nursing makes to patient care in the way they think about patient problems. In the case study relating to Bill, we have seen that he is able to recover partially through the application of a plan, agreed with Bill, to fulfil the needs identified in Gillian's nursing diagnosis. The nursing process, including diagnosis, offers practitioners a chance to reflect and gives them directions for doing so, which is particularly helpful to the novice practitioner (Wilson et al., 2018).

Conversely, problems which may arise from such systematic thinking are that patients may feel they are being 'processed' rather than being viewed as individuals with unique needs. Gillian might have spent her first meeting with Bill completing paperwork instead and firing questions at him. This might also have made Bill feel like he was being 'processed'. Avoiding the conveyor belt approach to nursing assessment and diagnosis is all about establishing a rapport with patients such that they become a part of the process, dictating at least some of the content of the diagnosis and subsequent plan according to their preferences and abilities.

When nurses are reliant on a process, it can also sometimes be difficult for them to think creatively and differently about their patient's problems and identify innovative solutions. Gillian identified one creative solution – Bill getting involved with his local church group again, as well as a Cruse support group – as a foundation for developing interaction. Read the following case study and then complete Activity 5.3 in order to identify some other potential benefits and problems with establishing a nursing diagnosis.

Case study: Jon's spiritual needs

Jon is a 10-year-old boy with leukaemia. He has had radiotherapy and a bone marrow transplant, but these have been unsuccessful. He is now having chemotherapy, which he is finding very tiring. Jon's mother, Angie, is staying with him in the hospital, where he has been admitted because his blood count is low. Angie is exhausted and finds it really difficult to talk to Jon about his illness as she knows his prognosis is poor and she cannot hide her distress from him. Jon knows his mother is distressed but cannot talk to her about it because she shuts him out by talking about 'childish' things. Jon confides his concern for his mother to Bisrat, an older nurse working in the children's cancer unit and someone whom Jon trusts. Jon says that he knows he is going to die and that everyone dies eventually anyway, so why hide from it? What he is finding hard is that no one seems to want to talk to him about it and they are always trying to 'jolly him along'. Jon has so many ideas and questions that he is looking to have answered. Bisrat identifies that Jon has unmet spiritual needs. She sits down with him and asks him what he wants to know. Jon asks what will happen to him at the end and if he will be in pain. Bisrat tells him that he will become more and more tired and eventually slip into unconsciousness. Jon asks if this is like sleeping, but Bisrat is careful to make the distinction between sleep and unconsciousness so that Jon is not concerned to go to sleep at night. She suggests Jon starts keeping a diary so that he can record his thoughts and feelings. Bisrat says that this might help him when he finds the right time to talk with his mum, but in the meantime Bisrat is happy to talk with him whenever she is working. Jon asks what will happen to his things when he dies, and Bisrat tells him they will be given to his mother. Jon thinks about this for a long time and then says that his diary can be a present to his mum.

Over the next week, Jon writes and draws in his diary, and at the end of the week Bisrat finds Jon and Angie talking quietly. Angie later comes to find Bisrat to thank her for helping her and Jon. She says that Jon's acceptance of his illness has helped to calm some of her own fears. The other nurses ask Bisrat what she did as they have noticed a change in the relationship between Jon and his mother.

Jon gradually deteriorates and Bisrat is now assigned to his care each time she is working. Jon dies at the end of the following week. Bisrat gathers up his things and gives them to his mother, telling her that the diary was a special present from Jon to her.

Activity 5.3   Critical thinking

Read the case study about Jon again and identify the potential benefits of the nursing diagnosis for Jon, for Bisrat and for other professionals. What might be the potential consequences for Jon's mother? Then consider any potential problems that the nursing diagnosis might create for the same group of people.

Having read Jon's case study, think about patients you have recently met on placement. Through reflection, how would you develop a nursing diagnosis of their spiritual needs? Which of the 6Cs does this relate to?

An outline answer is given at the end of the chapter.

Spirituality is often the section in patient assessment that is left blank or completed incorrectly in terms of focusing only on religious beliefs. However, spirituality is much more than this in terms of how people perceive themselves existing in the universe and have a sense of being (Clarke, 2013). Research suggests that spiritual distress is a meaningful and useful nursing diagnosis and therefore nurses would do well to better understand it (Caldeira et al., 2017). Being able to explain to others the characteristics of the nursing diagnosis and how you are using it also includes risk-assessing it in terms of the potential benefits and problems.

In the case study, Jon and Angie have benefited from Bisrat's creative thinking resulting from her accurate and insightful nursing diagnosis. However, there are also risks attached because Bisrat only has a snapshot view of their relationship and Jon's maturity of understanding. Bisrat's good communication skills helped to support her development of the nursing diagnosis as well as its problem-solving, finding a solution and plan for implementation.

From having looked at some of the particular benefits and problems that establishing a nursing diagnosis can pose, you should now be ready to start to develop nursing diagnoses yourself using a patient assessment.

Developing a nursing diagnosis from a patient assessment

Carpenito-Moyet (2016) identifies a number of different categories of nursing diagnosis. These include:

- actual – the diagnosis is supported by the presence of major defining characteristics such as verbalisation of the inability to cope;
- risk – identifying vulnerability to the problem, such as risk of carer strain;
- possible diagnosis – there are cues for a possible problem, but further information is needed to confirm this (e.g. non-compliance might be an informed autonomous decision or might relate to lack of understanding);
- wellness – identifying the potential for being even better, such as managing health more effectively;
- syndrome diagnosis – a number of nursing diagnoses relate to a specific event (e.g. domestic violence may give rise to a number of different nursing diagnoses, but these all relate to a specific event); and
- diagnostic cluster – these are nursing diagnoses that relate to particular patient group situations, such as standard post-procedure care (e.g. following an endoscopy).

In order to assess the patient, you will need to collect and interpret information (for more detail on this, return to Chapter 3). This will include:

- medical history;
- history of the current problem;
- how the patient is feeling; and
- patient understanding of the problem.

All of these contribute to you being able to establish a nursing diagnosis. You will also need to think about psychological, physiological, sociocultural, spiritual and environmental factors, as well as the skills you need to deploy in relation to communication, analysis, creative thinking and problem-solving. Consider the following case study and then complete Activity 5.4.

Case study: Mabel's accident

Mabel is 56 years old and lives with a learning disability. She lives in the community in a supported living house. Mabel was crossing the road and got hit by a car that did not stop. Mabel was found unconscious by a cyclist, who called an ambulance and stayed with her until it arrived.

Mabel wakes up in the ambulance but remains groggy and confused. Her Glasgow Coma Scale (GCS) score is 13. She has a headache and vomits once before reaching the hospital. Mabel is medically diagnosed with a head injury and admitted to the trauma ward.

When admitted to the trauma ward, Mabel becomes agitated by the strange environment and lashes out. She stays in the ward one night for observation and to receive anti-sickness medication and analgesia for her headache. When Mabel is discharged, she is given head injury advice and told to come back if her symptoms worsen. This is repeated to the care worker who comes to collect Mabel.

Activity 5.4   Critical thinking

After reading the case study, think about and list the different nursing diagnoses you can develop for Mabel. What categories do they fit with? What are the defining characteristics?

An outline answer is given at the end of the chapter.

You will have identified the possible nursing diagnoses as fitting into each of the categories described earlier. It might have been harder to think about the terms in which you wanted to describe them. Have a look at the diagnoses laid out in Carpenito-Moyet (2016) to help you with this.

Conclusion

Nursing diagnoses offer a nursing perspective on the problems that patients present with and can be focused on just the nursing elements or in collaboration with other professionals, but always in collaboration with the patient when they have the capacity to be involved. They articulate what expert nurses do all the time, and therefore are especially useful for those who are less experienced in practice. Nursing diagnoses are systematic and the starting point for any subsequent care planning. Therefore, they need to be accurately defined so that they are universally understood.

Chapter summary

This chapter has explained what a nursing diagnosis is and where it is placed in the nursing process, as well as offering some examples of different nursing diagnoses. It has clarified some of the advantages and disadvantages of using nursing diagnoses, as well as some of the potential problems they may pose for the patient and the nurse. You have been challenged to begin to think about your definition of what nursing is and what nurses do in order to contribute to advancing your professional understanding. You have been invited, through the activities, to apply critical thinking to the development of nursing diagnoses in different situations. They are the starting point for planning care; these themes will be revisited in Chapter 9.

Activities: brief outline answers

Activity 5.1   Reflection (page 79)

You might have formulated patients' problems and needs according to their medical diagnosis, what information was handed over to you and what patients said. Terminology is therefore likely to have varied. Care plans that contain vague diagnoses are difficult to work with. For example, what does limited mobility mean? At what blood sugar level does a particular person living with diabetes start to suffer the effects of hypoglycaemia? What level of help does an elderly person need with their washing and dressing? Do the care plan and nursing diagnosis make this clear, or does everyone new to their care have to ask the person each time?

Activity 5.2   Reflection (page 81)

You may have initially thought that nursing was about caring for people, although you could not really define this other than supporting patients who are feeling unwell by making them as comfortable as possible. You might also have identified nursing as giving medications. You could have been informed by the media and some of the programme dramas about nurses. You may also have based your definition on personal experience of being a patient. You are likely to realise now that nursing is based on the diagnoses that nurses make, which determine their nursing actions. While care is a key principle in any action taken by nurses, you need to be able to articulate your nursing diagnosis in order to explain your actions. What will have informed this conclusion is your placement experiences of seeing other nurses in action and being a novice nurse yourself. This is further informed by your learning theoretical elements such as accountability and the principles of the 6Cs. Nursing is therefore about recognising the uniqueness of each person and their needs and developing a nursing diagnosis that directs nursing actions to help individuals attain their health potential.

Activity 5.3 Critical thinking (page 86)

You might have identified the benefits of this nursing diagnosis as making sure that Jon's needs are respected and acknowledged by him receiving honest answers to his questions. In addition, the relationship between him and his mother is improved through the diary, stimulating discussion about his spiritual needs. The potential benefits for Jon's mother include having a lasting memento from Jon, feeling supported and a reduction in her anxiety. The benefits to Jon's nurse, Bisrat, are that she is able to identify Jon's individual need in addition to that of his medical diagnosis of leukaemia and deterioration.

The potential problems you might have identified are the risk of further alienation between Jon and his mother and that the diary could increase her pain after his death through what Jon has written. The potential problem for the nurse is in accurately gauging Jon's mental maturity to be able to understand and deal with the truth of his dying. The problem for other professionals may be in understanding Bisrat's reasoning processes. Documenting her reasoning using the standardised care plan and clear terms could be helpful in supporting other professionals' understanding. The most relevant core values from the 6Cs here are courage, care and compassion.

Activity 5.4 Critical thinking (page 88)

You could have identified an actual diagnosis of a lack of understanding and communication issues, which may be a result of Mabel's learning disability, the trauma or a mixture of both. This would have been evident from the responses Mabel gave. You might also have identified a syndrome diagnosis of head injury, which included the headache and nausea that Mabel was complaining of. You might have considered a risk diagnosis for communication and how to ensure that Mabel understood the head injury guidance given. The defining characteristics of these diagnoses, according to Carpenito-Moyet (2016), would be as follows:

- nausea – wave-like sensation with salivation, pallor and tachycardia, subjective descriptions;
- confusion – disorientation, fear and anxiety;
- pain – the patient reports and describes the sensation and intensity of painful stimuli; and
- congruence between verbal and non-verbal message.

Further reading

Ackley, BJ, Ladwig, GB, Makic, MB, Martinez-Kratz, M and Zanotti, M (2022) *Nursing Diagnosis Handbook E-Book: An Evidence-Based Guide to Planning Care* (12th edn). St Louis: Elsevier.

A great tool for looking in detail at assessment, diagnosis and care planning.

Carpenito-Moyet, LJ (2016) *Handbook of Nursing Diagnosis* (15th edn). Philadelphia, PA: Wolters Kluwer Health/Lippincott Williams Wilkins.

This book identifies the history of nursing diagnosis and some of the issues nurses have with the concept, and sets out in detail the features and characteristics of a variety of nursing diagnoses. It is especially useful for the novice practitioner.

Useful websites

www.nanda.org

This website contains the NANDA nursing diagnoses guidelines and updated information.

https://nurse.org/resources/nursing-diagnosis-guide/#the-4-types-of-nursing-diagnoses

A valuable guide to all things about nursing diagnoses.

Chapter 6

Principles of care planning

Peter Ellis

NMC Future Nurse: Standards of Proficiency for Registered Nurses

This chapter will address the following platforms and proficiencies:

Platform 1: Being an accountable professional

At the point of registration, the registered nurse will be able to:

1.2 understand and apply relevant legal, regulatory and governance requirements, policies, and ethical frameworks, including any mandatory reporting duties, to all areas of practice, differentiating where appropriate between the devolved legislatures of the United Kingdom.

Platform 3: Assessing needs and planning care

At the point of registration, the registered nurse will be able to:

3.4 understand and apply a person-centred approach to nursing care, demonstrating shared assessment, planning, decision making and goal setting when working with people, their families, communities and populations of all ages.

3.7 understand and apply the principles and processes for making reasonable adjustments.

3.8 understand and apply the relevant laws about mental capacity for the country in which you are practising when making decisions in relation to people who do not have capacity.

3.15 demonstrate the ability to work in partnership with people, families and carers to continuously monitor, evaluate and reassess the effectiveness of all agreed nursing care plans and care, sharing decision making and readjusting agreed goals, documenting progress and decisions made.

3.16 demonstrate knowledge of when and how to refer people safely to other professionals or services for clinical intervention or support.

Platform 5: Leading and managing nursing care and working in teams

At the point of registration, the registered nurse will be able to:

5.4 demonstrate an understanding of the roles, responsibilities and scope of practice of all members of the nursing and interdisciplinary team and how to make best use of the contributions of others involved in providing care.

5.9 demonstrate the ability to challenge and provide constructive feedback about care delivered by others in the team, and help them to identify and agree individual learning needs.

Chapter aims

After reading this chapter, you will be able to:

- explain the purpose of care plans;
- identify a nursing problem;
- understand the stages of care planning;
- make the connection between nursing as a therapy and nursing care outcomes; and
- develop a care plan.

Introduction

Case study: Grace's loss of confidence

Grace is 78 years old and lives with her friend, Mary, in a semi-detached house. She suffered a fall recently that has knocked her confidence. Grace is normally an outgoing individual, having previously attended many activities such as a reading group and helping out at a local lunch club, but she is now scared to leave the house alone. Mary has severe arthritis and has not been able to help Grace much. Siobhan, a nurse working with the intermediate care team, picks up Grace's referral and assesses Grace's needs and plans her care. The first thing she observes when visiting Grace at home is that there are many loose rugs downstairs and that the stairs leading up to her first-floor bedroom are rather steep, with only the main banister for support. There is also a step from the kitchen into the dining area. When Siobhan questions Grace about her eyesight, Grace admits that this has become progressively worse because of her diabetes. Siobhan checks Grace's blood sugar reading and the medication she is taking. The blood sugar reading is within normal limits.

(Continued)

(Continued)

When Siobhan questions Grace about what led to her fall, Grace breaks down and says she and Mary had had a row about cooking supper, and she was not looking where she was going and tripped and fell. She felt unhappy and depressed, and this had worsened since the fall as she did not feel safe going out, but missed her other friends.

Siobhan identifies that Grace has issues with an unsafe environment and her mobility, as well as psychosocial issues that need to be factored into a plan of care. Working with Grace, Siobhan is able to develop a plan of care that includes other professionals such as the occupational therapist to ensure that Grace gets the adaptation aids which will make the house safer, the advice which will empower her to manage to self-care, and psychological support which will help address her low mood. Because Siobhan works closely with other professionals such as the occupational therapists in the intermediate care team, she is able to share her care plan and discuss some of the planned interventions.

Grace's house had an extra handrail fitted to the stairs and a wall-mounted grab rail fitted by the kitchen step. Grace and Mary asked a friend to remove the loose rugs and Grace invited people from the lunch club to visit her. The next time Siobhan saw Grace, she appeared more confident and happier.

This chapter builds on the previous ones by considering the elements that need to be written into care planning in order to ensure a holistic and person-centred application of the nursing process. A complete nursing care plan is also helpful for other professionals to understand how nursing actions fit with their priorities for the care of an individual. The case study above illustrates how teams work together and can involve different professionals in planning interventions for their patients. It also highlights how the principles of communication, care and commitment – three of the 6Cs – are enacted. This chapter will explain why care plans are needed and how to determine nursing interventions. Through the activities, you will be given the opportunity to make the connection between nursing as a therapy and nursing care outcomes and to develop a written care plan.

Why care plans are needed

Support and care planning is necessary because patients' needs are greater than just their medical needs, and therefore will involve different professionals. Creating a personalised care plan can offer benefits for patients, health and social care professionals, and the organisations within which they work. Some of these benefits include:

- personalised care – involving patients in deciding what their needs are and how these might be met;
- holistic care – care that considers all of the physical, psychological, social and spiritual elements of care a patient needs;

- promoting health – exploring patients' understanding of their problem and providing information as needed to help people achieve a higher level of wellness;
- reducing health inequalities – standardising care helps organisations to share and disseminate good practice;
- stimulating choice – the choices patients make can inform commissioning decisions; and
- reducing inefficiency – resources are deployed and used according to needs.

(Department of Health, 2009)

Perhaps the biggest reason that care plans are important is that they are used to pass the care of the patient from one professional to another in a way that ensures the individual's needs can be clearly understood by all concerned. This ability to coordinate care between professionals is known as continuity of care, which is said to positively impact on people's well-being and enable them to achieve the outcomes identified in their care plan (National Institute for Health and Care Excellence, NICE, 2019). Consider the following case study to see how these benefits might be achieved in practice and then answer the questions in Activity 6.1.

Case study: Lenny's long-term mental health condition

Lenny had started to hide in his room because he was hearing voices and thought his girlfriend, Milly, was trying to kill him. Milly became scared of Lenny and asked their GP, Paul, for help. Paul came to the house and spoke to Lenny through the door of his room. He could see that Lenny was in need of help but could not coax him out of his room. Lenny was admitted to the local mental health unit under the Mental Health Act 1983, which allows his detention in a hospital even if it is against Lenny's will, on the grounds of keeping him and others safe from harm. The fact that Lenny had started to become violent towards Milly made the admission necessary. Milly found all of this terribly upsetting and left Lenny at this time.

When Lenny was first admitted, his nurse, Moira, noted that he was confused, angry and scared. Moira understood Lenny's need to feel safe and gave him time and space to adjust. She showed Lenny to his room and asked him if he wanted something to drink. Knowing that Lenny was likely to be suspicious of any drink she made for him, Moira got a plastic bottle of Coke from the vending machine and gave it to Lenny unopened. Moira proceeded to talk to Lenny about his likes and dislikes over the next few days – when he liked to go to bed and get up, what activities he enjoyed, and so on. In this way, Moira started to build a therapeutic relationship with him as she ensured Lenny's preferences were taken into account, thereby giving Lenny as much control over his life as possible given the circumstances.

(Continued)

(Continued)

Lenny had been prescribed medication to help his symptoms. Moira was the nurse who had the most success in getting him to take it. Moira also managed to persuade Lenny to eat a proper meal by removing the things he had told her he did not like, such as cabbage and similar vegetables. Moira also managed to persuade Lenny to wash some days by telling him that she would stand guard at the door to make sure no one came into the bathroom while he was doing so.

Gradually, as Lenny started to respond to the medication and gain some sense of normality, Moira was able to explain what had happened to him and what could be done to keep his symptoms under control. When planning his care, Moira asked Lenny what he wanted to happen. When looking at his discharge planning, Lenny said that he could not go back to where he had previously lived because since his girlfriend had left, the rent had lapsed and the flat had new tenants. Moira suggested speaking to the social worker, who could help Lenny look at the options available to him.

Lenny met with the social worker, Jim, and a discharge plan was formulated that found Lenny some space in a halfway hostel for people with mental health issues. Moira helped Lenny to organise what he needed to take to the hostel. Moira also identified where Lenny could seek help if he needed it and explained his medication prior to discharge, and the importance of continuing to take it even though he felt well. Lenny was discharged to the halfway hostel, where he met up with Peter, his community mental health nurse, who would be continuing his care. With the help of Peter and Jim, Lenny eventually managed to secure some part-time work in a local supermarket.

The case study illustrates Moira offering Lenny choices in what he eats and personalising his care by meeting his needs for privacy. She also waits until he is ready to hear the explanation of his condition so that he can be more informed on how he can stay healthy. Only when Lenny's medication has started to have a therapeutic effect does Moira involve Jim, the social worker, to find Lenny work and somewhere to live. People with mental health problems suffer many inequalities, not least in the job market, and it is therefore important to set Lenny up to succeed. The choice of accommodation is also limited, but the halfway hostel recognises Lenny's stage of recovery and is used to people with mental health issues. Other housing options might not be as understanding. Inclusion of the community mental health nurse is a good use of resources in seeking to help Lenny stay well in the community and prevent a quick return to the mental health unit, supporting him in employment and in the longer term. You will find more information about the Mental Health Act 1983 under 'Useful websites' at the end of the chapter.

Completing Activity 6.1 will help you to think about the benefits of care planning in other settings.

Activity 6.1   Critical thinking

Think about the next placement you are going to. Make a list of questions about why care plans are needed in that setting and how they are used. Consider how health inequalities might be reduced by using personalised care plans in that setting.

An outline answer is given at the end of the chapter.

Modern health and social care tries to include patients in their own care wherever possible. Patients' involvement has become enshrined in government health policy since the 1990s and it is considered good practice to include patients in decisions made about their care and is a commitment the NHS makes to patients (NHS, ND). In fact, the Mental Capacity Act 2005 specifically states that 'a person must be assumed to have capacity unless it is established that he lacks capacity' and 'a person is not to be treated as unable to make a decision unless all practicable steps to help him to do so have been taken without success'. What this essentially means is that where anybody has the ability (capacity) to make choices, they should be helped to do so; this is especially important when decisions are being made that affect their care.

Activity 6.2   Reflection

Think about an occasion when you, or someone you love, engaged with health or social care services. Consider how you, or they, were made to feel about their level of involvement in the decisions being made about care. How well was this done and how did it make you/them feel?

As this activity is based on your experience, there is no outline answer at the end of the chapter.

Consequently, when you are thinking about why care plans are needed, your answer might be because they can demonstrate inclusion of the patient's priorities and needs, and the planning process undertaken with the patient. They also show respect for the person as an autonomous being. The next step to consider is how patients' priorities can be translated into nursing problems.

Identifying a nursing problem

We have already touched upon some nursing problems in Chapter 5 when looking at nursing diagnoses. The intention here is to look more closely at what is considered a nursing problem and how you can interpret this as part of the care planning process.

Nursing problems are quite simply those care problems that have a nursing context. As you will have seen highlighted in Chapter 5, nursing problems can be used to develop nursing diagnoses, but they need to use standardised language that is easily understood by both professionals and patients. For example, a patient has unmet informational needs about his medical diagnosis, which is causing anxiety. When you are identifying the nursing problem, this does not mean imposing your nursing viewpoint. Instead, it means working with the patient to establish caring priorities. The caring priority in this example would be to ensure that the patient understands the medical diagnosis and its implications in order to take an active and informed part in what happens next, assuming that is what they choose to do.

Therefore, identifying a nursing problem involves utilising the communication skills that you will have identified in Chapter 3 in order to develop a therapeutic relationship where you are able to demonstrate having a *sympathetic presence*. This means being able to understand your patient's needs in a person-centred way and working with the core values of the 6Cs in ways that are meaningful to the patient and which advance nursing care and practice. In practice, this means engaging with care planning that is based on patient preference rather than only your professional opinion. When patient preferences are aligned with nurses' care priorities, nursing care can be improved as well as patient outcomes including their safety (Ringdal et al., 2017).

Activity 6.3   Reflection

Look back at the case study involving Lenny and his nurse, Moira. Consider how Moira demonstrated her engagement with the 6Cs when planning Lenny's care in a person-centred manner.

An outline answer is given at the end of the chapter.

One way in which you can identify the nursing problem is to use the think-aloud reasoning process, which might involve the patient, as appropriate, as well as other professionals (Funkesson et al., 2007). This process identifies the nursing knowledge you are using to explain how the problem has been formulated while at the same time also taking note of the patient experience and contribution. The think-aloud process enables everyone involved to voice what they are thinking as the process progresses (Burbach et al., 2015), which enables the resulting plan to represent an amalgamation of the views of everyone involved.

When you are aligning nursing problems with patient problems, you are working in a person-centred way so that the care planning process is also person-centred. Person-centred understanding here is based on McCormack and McCance's (2016) way of looking at problems from the person's perspective and empowering the patient to make autonomous decisions. The involvement of other professionals and the patient in the process will also add to the holistic credentials of the plan that is being made (as we saw in the case studies involving Grace and Lenny). Reading the next case study will help you to understand how to identify nursing problems in a person-centred way.

Case study: David's anxiety about having a vaccination

David is 15 years old and at secondary school. He is due to have his BCG injection (a vaccination against tuberculosis), and all the teenagers in his year queue in the school hall, where they are seen by the school nurse, Fiona, for the injection. David is unwilling to have the injection and will not cooperate. He becomes more and more distressed and then walks out, knocking a stack of papers to the floor on his way past.

Fiona decides to talk to David alone later. She meets David in her office the next day and asks him how he is feeling. David tells her that he felt very angry yesterday because he had had a row with his mum at home following the letter sent home from school about the impending injection. David's mum had told him how important it was for him to have this injection and David had told her that he did not understand why he needed it. He found it difficult queuing for the injection and started to feel more and more stressed as he waited with his peers. David described how his heart was racing and he broke out in a cold sweat when approaching the desk where Fiona was giving the injection. He did not want to show himself up in front of his mates and decided it was better to walk out. He did not see the point in having the injection as he did not mix with anyone who was sick and he did not think it was worth the hassle.

Fiona explained to David why the injection was important. She also asked him whether he had ever had any unpleasant experiences with injections. David said that he could remember going to his doctor with his mother as a young child and the nurse talking kindly to him and then putting what felt like a nail in his bottom. He had never forgotten it, and whenever he was now approached by health professionals he was very distrustful. Fiona explained that she thought David's anxiety had produced his feeling of panic and psychological unease. Fiona talked David through the injection process, the risks and benefits, and offered for David to have the injection in private. She talked through some visualisation techniques with David to help control some of his anxiety. David felt calmer and more in control, and asked Fiona to give him the injection now. He practised the techniques that she had taught him while Fiona gave the injection, and he hardly felt anything. Fiona advised David to talk to his mum about this in case his anxiety recurred in the future.

This case study demonstrates how *sympathetic presence* is part of a non-judgemental attitude that is essential for building trust and rapport. The case study can also be related to the core value of compassion by taking note of how patients are feeling and being with them. It would have been easy for Fiona to have made a judgement that David was behaving like a *typical teenager* who did not want to be told what to do. However, she realised that there was a problem underlying his behaviour – anxiety – which could be managed as a nursing problem of anxiety due to lack of understanding and fear of pain. By offering information to aid David's understanding, as well as some techniques, such as visualisation distraction, where the person thinks of something pleasant and a calm context in which they have previously been happy, Fiona and David managed to work together, with the outcome of David having the injection. However, Fiona recognises that David's anxiety could recur. By asking him to talk to his mum about it, Fiona is helping David to enlist further support and demonstrating commitment to him through seeking future solutions.

Nursing problems are not always issues that can be dealt with and resolved at the present time. They may require more long-term management going forward. For this reason, it is important to recognise that within the care planning process there will be short- as well as medium- and long-term goals. We will now examine the stages of the care planning process in more detail.

The stages of care planning

The main stages of the nursing process have already been illustrated in Chapter 5 (see Figure 5.1, page 83). The stages of care planning follow the nursing process in a similar cyclical way, as follows:

1. identifying the problem and nursing diagnosis – clearly defining what these are from patient assessment information and discussion with the person;

2. establishing the goals – clearly defined benchmarks for measuring achievement of problem-solving that have been agreed with the person;

3. determining nursing interventions – listing nurses' actions based on assessed understanding of the situation and your knowledge and expertise;

4. evaluation of care processes – documenting outcomes of the care given; and

5. review dates – the date by which it is expected that a change will have been effected.

The application of the stages is identified in the box below.

As previously mentioned, it is important that you consider short-, medium- and long-term goals as well as psychosocial, spiritual and physical concerns in order for the care planning process to be holistic. The stages listed above are easy to recognise within certain fields of nursing, such as within hospital wards; however, they may not be so obvious within the documentation used in ambulatory care areas or the community. Nevertheless, these processes are part of nurses' care planning thinking, no matter where they work, and therefore it is important to be clear about how this is taking place in order to be able to share the rationale for the decisions you have made about the care of your patient (you can read more on decision-making in care planning in Chapter 9). We will now translate some of these principles into developing a written care plan.

Stages of the care planning process

Stage 1

The patient may have more than one problem, particularly in complex cases. The order in which the problems are identified will be determined by the nursing model (see Chapter 7) you are using to frame the patient assessment and care planning process as well as the patient's current dependency. Problems will also be actual as well as potential because the care planning process includes risk-assessing and managing potential problems. In nursing care planning, it is important to be clear as to why a problem is a nursing problem. For example, patient anxiety is a nursing problem because nursing is about making patients feel listened to, comfortable, informed, and psychologically and socially safe.

Stage 2

The goal is what the patient will be able to do, or perhaps how they will feel, at the end of a care process (e.g. be able to walk with one stick or feel less anxious). Goals need to be specific, measurable, achievable, relevant and time-based (i.e. SMART). If goals are too vague, it will be difficult to assess progress or to sustain motivation. Goals also need to be short-, medium- and long-term, as previously described. Another criterion that can be used when formulating goals is the PRODUCT criteria, described by Wilson et al. (2018) as patient-centred, recordable, observable and measurable, directive, understandable and clear, credible, and time-related. There are clear similarities between the SMART and PRODUCT criteria in that they need to be agreed with the patient and clear and measurable within a particular time span. Which one you use will depend on the best fit with the patient and context of care.

Stage 3

Determining nursing interventions is about giving specific instructions about what you think nurses need to do in order to address the problem identified and reach the specific goal. Nursing interventions should also be evidence-based (Ellis, 2023) and, where available, use the latest research (Wilson et al., 2018). They should also incorporate the patient or service user's preferences and individual needs, such as cultural needs. Nursing interventions also need to be realistic and sustainable within the resources available.

(Continued)

(Continued)

Stage 4

When evaluating, it is necessary to revisit the problem definitions and goal statements in order to identify any changes that have occurred as well as any modifications that need to be made. Resolution of the problem may not always occur completely, and therefore ongoing care may require refining and modifying the definition of the problem and the planned nursing interventions.

Stage 5

The review dates need to be set within a realistic timescale for potential resolution of the particular problem. These are also important for communication between teams and continuity of care. These will ensure that there are particular checkpoints for evaluating a patient's progress and the outcome of care processes. This is also important to make sure that resources are used efficiently and appropriately.

Developing a written care plan

Caring for patients requires a clear vision of what you hope to achieve, who is to carry out the prescribed nursing interventions, and how these are progressing (Wilson et al., 2018). An example care plan that includes the stages described above can be found in the box below and Table 6.1.

Example care plan

Tim's assessment

Tim has been admitted to day surgery for a haemorrhoidectomy. Tim is a 50-year-old firefighter who works shifts that include days and nights. He lives in a semi-detached house with his wife, Carol, and three children, aged 8, 12 and 14 years old. They have no pets. Carol also works shifts as a registered nurse. Tim is a non-smoker and only drinks alcohol on his days off duty. Tim's body mass index is 24. On admission, Tim's vital signs are temperature 36.2°C, pulse 74 bpm, respirations 12 breaths/minute and blood pressure 122/82 mmHg. Tim will have his operation under general anaesthetic. He is expected to make a sufficient recovery to be able to go home later today after his surgery and be cared for by his wife.

Some common problems with writing care plans are now provided in the following case studies to help you think about how you might avoid them. Activities 6.4 and 6.5 ask you to think critically about the problems and possible solutions.

Problem	Goal	Nursing interventions	Evaluation	Review date
Anxiety that the operation will have an impact on his ability to work	*Short-term*: Tim's Hospital Anxiety and Depression Scale (HADS) measurement is within the normal range by the time he is discharged from day surgery. *Long-term*: Tim is able to work after 14 days' rest.	The registered nurse will give Tim time and space to express his anxieties before and after his surgery. The registered nurse will provide Tim with information about the procedure and likely effects before the operation and at the point of discharge from day surgery. The registered nurse will advise Tim when he is being discharged from day surgery of the precautions to take to avoid complications. The registered nurse will check Tim's anxiety using the HADS prior to surgery and prior to discharge, and will communicate the results to the team.	Tim expressed his concerns about getting back to work and being able to do what he did before. The operation has been explained to Tim by the surgeon and the registered nurse, and he understands that he will not be able to undertake firefighting duties for 14 days. Tim has been advised of the need to avoid constipation and of the signs of infection. Tim has been given the out-of-hours number for day surgery.	Before discharge
Post-operative pain and nausea	*Short-term*: Tim's pain and nausea will be controlled with post-operative medication. *Long-term*: Tim will not have any pain or nausea after 14 days.	The registered nurse will check Tim's pain and nausea score (using numerical rating scales) on return from surgery, 30 minutes after giving any medication or an hour following his return from surgery and prior to discharge. The registered nurse/nursing associate will position Tim comfortably. The registered nurse will ensure that Tim has pain medication to take home and understands how to take it. The registered nurse will instruct Tim and his wife where to seek further help if his pain or nausea worsens when he is at home.	Tim's pain score on return from surgery was 3 and his nausea score was 1. He was given prescribed pain and nausea medication by the registered nurse, which alleviated his symptoms as measured 30 minutes after administration. By the time he was discharged, Tim's pain and nausea scores were 0. Tim and his wife understood how to take his medication and that he could not drink alcohol or operate machinery while taking it.	On return from theatre, 30 minutes after administering medication, at one-hour post-return from theatre and on discharge

(Continued)

Table 6.1 (Continued)

Problem	Goal	Nursing interventions	Evaluation	Review date
Cognitive ability and orientation to time and place	*Short-term*: Tim will be fully oriented to time and place on discharge.	The registered nurse/nursing associate will give Tim time to wake up slowly.	Tim was sleepy on his return to the ward from theatre, with a sedation score of 3. He did ask twice what the time was. On discharge, Tim was fully oriented to time and place, although he still felt a bit tired, and was therefore advised to rest when he got home.	On return from theatre
		The registered nurse/nursing associate will tell Tim that he has returned to the ward and what the time is.		
	Long-term: Tim will be able to process decision-making information cognitively after 24 hours.	The registered nurse will check Tim's sedation score using the Ramsay Sedation Scale.		
		The registered nurse will offer explanations when Tim is fully awake.		
Actual problem: Surgical rectal wound	Wound shows signs of healing and absence of infection by end of week 1.	The registered nurse will observe the wound for any bleeding post-operatively prior to discharge.	Tim's wound showed some minimal bleeding on the pad. He was discharged with spare pads.	Before discharge
		The registered nurse will advise Tim how to care for the wound at home.		
Potential problem: Infection		The registered nurse will advise Tim and his wife of the signs of infection and to seek help from his GP if any of these occur.		
Long-term problem: Further haemorrhoids	Tim is maintaining a high-fibre diet by day 7.	The registered nurse/nursing associate advises Tim about high-fibre diet options and drinking at least 2 litres of water per day.	On discharge from day surgery, Tim knew what dietary and fluid options were helpful for his recovery.	On discharge

Table 6.1 Example care plan (see also the box on page 102)

Case study: Setting goals for Mindi

Mindi has diabetes and a chest infection. The student nurse looking after her has identified a number of problems, one of which is maintaining blood glucose control. She writes the goal as 'able to maintain normal blood glucose levels'.

Activity 6.4   Critical thinking

Can you identify any problems with this as a goal when applying SMART principles?

An outline answer is given at the end of the chapter.

Case study: Prescribing nursing interventions for George

George has had a stroke. He has recovered some of his speech but remains immobile. He is very depressed and finds it difficult to accept that other people need to carry out his care needs. The student nurse looking after George plans the following nursing interventions:

- Give all care to George.
- Refer to a counsellor.
- Refer to the occupational therapist.
- Refer to the physiotherapist.
- Complete an anxiety and depression scale score.

Activity 6.5   Critical thinking

Can you identify any problems with these nursing interventions?

An outline answer is given at the end of the chapter.

Activity 6.5 will help you to reflect on what you have learned so far about care planning and how you can apply this knowledge in practice.

Activity 6.6   Reflection

What are the main points that you need to remember when developing a care plan? How should you formulate goals? How can you ensure that your care planning process is person-centred and includes core values from the 6Cs as appropriate?

An outline answer is given at the end of the chapter.

The connection between nursing therapy and nursing care outcomes

Nursing seeks to support patients emotionally, psychologically, socially, spiritually and physically. As a nurse, you will need to find ways of being *with* the patient that enable you to develop a therapeutic relationship and a *sympathetic presence*, which means patients feel you understand their point of view. But at the same time, you also need to work systematically to achieve agreed goals. Nursing is reflected 'not in what we do, but in the way we provide care' (Hawkey and Williams, 2007, page 8).

Nurses have the greatest contact time with patients, and it is in how we use that contact time that nursing becomes therapeutic rather than task-oriented. Nursing care outcomes are therefore centred on the person within the patient rather than a medical diagnosis (i.e. they are based on the person's experience of care and recovery). Nevertheless, the professional background of staff involved with a care setting or patient will influence the approach to care planning and the way care is implemented (Worden and Challis, 2008). Concept mapping is one way in which it is possible to gain a holistic nursing view of the person rather than one based on a disease process model (Ogden et al., 2017). In concept mapping, assessment information is sorted into clusters to identify problem areas and consider relationships between them. This is a dynamic process that considers gaps in knowledge and information and develops understanding of the complexities of patients' situations. In this way, how you develop the therapeutic relationship with the patient can also be related to the nursing outcomes to assess the effectiveness of your care planning and nursing care.

Activity 6.7   Developing a care plan

On your next placement, try to use the principles introduced in this chapter to develop a care plan with your patient, and discuss it with your practice supervisor to see whether you have succeeded.

As this activity is based on your experience, there is no outline answer at the end of the chapter.

Conclusion

Person-centred care planning is based on developing a therapeutic relationship that recognises the person within the patient and concentrates on how care strategies are decided *with* – rather than *for* – that person. Care planning in this way will require you to nurture and develop your way of being with the patient rather than how we *do* nursing *to* them. In the busy health and social care environment, taking time with people may be difficult, but is also extremely rewarding in terms of achieving nursing outcomes and quality nursing care in line with the core values of the 6Cs.

Chapter summary

This chapter has explored why care planning is important for effective patient care. It has examined how the process of care planning relates to the nursing process and the different stages involved. You have been given the opportunity to avoid some of the pitfalls in care planning and to develop a care plan of your own. Consideration of how nursing therapy relates to nursing outcomes has promoted reflection on your nursing practice.

Activities: brief outline answers

Activity 6.1 Critical thinking (page 97)

The following questions will help you to identify why care plans are useful in a particular setting.

- What type of care plans are used here?
- How are care plans used?
- Do care plans follow the same format for each patient/condition?
- Are they based on a particular nursing model/philosophy?
- How do the staff record preferences and likes and dislikes?
- Are patients/carers always involved in the care plan or are there exceptions?
- If so, what are these exceptions?

Health inequalities might be reduced by considering how individual patient needs and planning might translate more widely and, for example, give patients living with mental health needs optimum chances and access to resources.

Activity 6.3 Reflection (page 98)

Care: Moira committed to helping Lenny in the best way she could and on his terms.

Compassion: Moira showed understanding and empathy and respected Lenny as a person, seeking to protect his dignity.

Competence: Moira understood how to approach Lenny's care needs in a timely fashion and involved others when needed.

Communication: Moira listened to Lenny and understood him. She communicated to him and to others who needed to be involved in his care.

Courage: Moira showed the ability to think laterally and tried different things to help Lenny, such as getting him a bottle of Coke and guarding the door while he bathed.

Commitment: Moira committed to support Lenny and used all her skills and knowledge to aid his recovery.

Activity 6.4   Critical thinking (page 105)

You might have questioned what is meant by normal, what is the time frame, and how this will be measured when writing an appropriate goal. You might have considered a better goal could be 'will maintain blood sugar levels between 5 and 8 mmol/L over the next seven days, measured by glucometer'. This sets out exactly the conditions to be measured and how this will be done.

Activity 6.5   Critical thinking (page 105)

You might have identified: first, these are not nursing interventions because many of them do not involve nurses; and second, there does not appear to be any involvement of George within these planned interventions. Therefore, nursing interventions might more appropriately include the following:

- Give George the time and space to express how he feels.
- Attentively listen to George to find out what his concerns and priorities are, and how he wishes to proceed with the way that he is cared for.
- Offer George some strategies for assisting with his care, and once these are determined add them to the plan of care.

This plan is more person-centred in its approach because it involves George in setting the priorities and in decision-making. While the referrals may be part of the care plan, they should not be the first solution because they are not in themselves nursing interventions.

Activity 6.6   Reflection (page 106)

You might have identified the importance of adopting a person-centred approach to assessment and care planning. This means identifying patient priorities and aligning these with nursing problems. You may have considered the different stages of care planning as identifying the problem and establishing goals that are specific, measurable, achievable, relevant and time-based. You might have considered that talking to patients, as well as giving them the time and space to express their needs and discuss care options and strategies, was an appropriate way to promote person-centred decision-making and implement working with the core values of the 6Cs.

Further reading

McCormack, B and McCance, T (2016) *Person-Centred Practice in Nursing and Health Care: Theory and Practice* (2nd edn). Oxford: Wiley-Blackwell.

This book offers a comprehensive and contemporaneous guide to person-centred nursing practice.

Wilson, B, Woollands, A and Barrett, D (2018) *Care Planning: A Guide for Nurses* (3rd edn). Harlow: Pearson Education.

This book gives a step-by-step guide to the care planning process and considers some nursing models that might frame it.

Useful websites

www.legislation.gov.uk/ukpga/2005/9/section/1

The Mental Capacity Act 2005 can be viewed here.

https://www.legislation.gov.uk/ukpga/1983/20/contents

The Mental Health Act 1983 can be viewed here. There are amendments made to this Act in the Mental Health Act 2007.

https://improve.bmj.com/person-centred-care-2/

A website dedicated to the idea of person-centred care from the *British Medical Journal.*

www.ombudsman.org.uk

This website contains a number of case studies about situations where care has been lacking, has not been person-centred or where it has gone wrong. Applying the principles of this chapter to those case studies might help you to understand the importance of care planning for better outcomes.

Chapter 7 Nursing models and care planning

Peter Ellis

NMC Future Nurse: Standards of Proficiency for Registered Nurses

This chapter will address the following platforms and proficiencies:

Platform 1: Being an accountable professional

At the point of registration, the registered nurse will be able to:

1.8 demonstrate the knowledge, skills and ability to think critically when applying evidence and drawing on experience to make evidence-informed decisions in all situations.

1.9 understand the need to base all decisions regarding care and interventions on people's needs and preferences, recognising and addressing any personal and external factors that may unduly influence their decisions.

1.16 demonstrate the ability to keep complete, clear, accurate and timely records.

Platform 2: Promoting health and preventing ill health

At the point of registration, the registered nurse will be able to:

2.10 provide information in accessible ways to help people understand and make decisions about their health, life choices, illness and care.

Platform 3: Assessing needs and planning care

At the point of registration, the registered nurse will be able to:

3.6 effectively assess a person's capacity to make decisions about their own care and to give or withhold consent.

3.15 demonstrate the ability to work in partnership with people, families and carers to continuously monitor, evaluate and reassess the effectiveness of all agreed nursing care plans and care, sharing decision making and readjusting agreed goals, documenting progress and decisions made.

3.16 demonstrate knowledge of when and how to refer people safely to other professionals or services for clinical intervention or support.

Platform 4: Providing and evaluating care

At the point of registration, the registered nurse will be able to:

4.2 work in partnership with people to encourage shared decision making in order to support individuals, their families and carers to manage their own care when appropriate.

Chapter aims

After reading this chapter, you will be able to:

- describe a variety of nursing models;
- identify the importance of nursing models;
- explain how the use of a nursing model can structure the assessment process; and
- describe how using a nursing model impacts on decision-making in care planning.

Introduction

Case study: Stella's asthma attack

Stella is a 50-year-old accountant who has suffered from bronchial asthma since childhood. Her job is pressured and can be stressful, particularly at certain times of the year when accounts need to be finalised for tax purposes. She takes medication for her asthma and has additional inhalers to use if she has an asthma attack.

It is autumn and the weather has become cold and damp. Stella had her flu vaccination two weeks ago as she was deemed to be at risk of becoming very ill with flu given her asthma. Yesterday, Stella woke up with a wheezy chest and her shortness of breath quite quickly became worse. She used her inhalers but they did not help. Her husband called an ambulance and Stella was admitted to hospital. Stella was admitted to the respiratory ward by Laura, who is a student nurse. Laura identified that the appropriate nursing model to frame Stella's assessment and care plan was Roper, Logan and Tierney's activities of daily living model, because this model helps to consider which areas of Stella's activity are compromised and how these might be improved. The model is also sufficiently systematic to ensure that areas which might at present not be compromised are also considered.

(Continued)

(Continued)

Laura assesses how Stella is currently compromised in the areas of daily living, including maintaining a safe environment, breathing, communication, controlling body temperature, eating and drinking, washing and dressing, mobilisation, expressing sexuality, death and dying, elimination, working and playing, and sleeping. She identifies that the greatest priorities at the moment are breathing, communication and mobility because Stella is short of breath. Laura's care planning therefore initially focuses on these areas and on nursing interventions that can be employed to help Stella. These include offering reassurance and explaining nursing actions, positioning Stella to aid her breathing, administering and monitoring the effects of prescribed medication, and undertaking nursing observations. When Stella's breathing improves, the nursing action will be to assist her to mobilise slowly and help her with personal hygiene needs. In terms of eating and drinking, the priority at the moment is to keep Stella hydrated.

Stella remained in hospital for a week, where she was treated for a chest infection. She was discharged and returned to work after a further two weeks.

Using a nursing model as a framework helps direct practitioners in the assessment and care planning process. As the case study above has illustrated, the choice of nursing model identifies areas to be assessed and gives direction for planning nursing interventions, particularly with regard to the focus of those interventions. This chapter will consider a number of nursing models and how they are used, and why they might be applied in different circumstances. It will also explore some of the main differences between the nursing models and how these relate to care planning. The chapter will also make the link between the nursing model and decisions made in the care planning process.

Why nursing models are important

There are different specialities of nursing, and therefore the way in which care is assessed, planned and delivered will vary between specialities. For example, nursing a patient with intensive care needs is different from nursing a patient in an ambulatory care environment, in the community or in a mental health setting. Equally, patients themselves are unique with their own differing needs. A one-size-fits-all model of nursing is therefore neither desirable nor practical, as it does not deal with the complexity of patients' health or personal needs or the nursing interventions needed to meet these needs. Nursing models were developed to reflect the nursing values and beliefs associated with nursing and to help express the focus and purpose of nursing activity with any individual patient with their unique nursing needs. Nursing models also identify how nursing priorities and concerns can be different from medicine (Wilson et al., 2018). While particular specialities may espouse certain nursing models, these models must always be aligned with the patient's presenting needs and wishes in order to ensure a person-centred and holistic assessment and care plan are achieved.

As a student moving between different specialities, you will come across a variety of models of nursing, some which are used in an obvious way and others not so. You will need to develop the ability to understand and apply these models seamlessly with different patients in different environments.

Completing Activity 7.1 will help you to think about why nursing models are important for the assessment and care planning process.

Activity 7.1   Reflection

Think about the nursing models you have seen used in practice. Consider the following questions:

- How did the model reflect the particular needs of the patient in the practice area?
- What was the impact of the model on the assessment and care planning process?
- If there was no nursing model in evidence, how were you able to justify what you were doing?
- How can you integrate working with nursing models and the 6Cs?

Although this activity is based on your experience, there is a limited outline answer at the end of the chapter.

It may sometimes appear that no nursing model is being used in a practice area because care pathway documentation is used instead. Care pathways (sometimes known as integrated care pathways, clinical pathways or patient pathways) are multidisciplinary because different professional groups can use them to record their activity with a patient and document their instructions and plans. Care pathways apply to a particular group of patients with similar problems. They often list specific criteria and actions (Wilson et al., 2018), such as those required to support a patient attending for routine, elective, surgery. Nevertheless, the framing of patient problems and evaluation of care will usually be based on the values and beliefs stemming from a particular nursing model. Therefore, what can on the surface appear to be working to a medical model by focusing on rectifying health deficits will often also be defined and underpinned by nursing principles based on the expertise of the practitioner – but only where the planning process takes account of the uniqueness of the individual patients. The continuing interest in the 6Cs means that these need to be considered in terms of how they are integrated into the application of the nursing model and the provision of care in ways that are meaningful. It is important to be clear how you describe and justify your nursing activity in order to communicate this accurately to the patient, as well as to other members of the nursing and interprofessional team as previously discussed.

Nursing models

Nursing models are based on the environment of care, the people involved in nursing activity, the health status of the patient, and the nursing capabilities and knowledge of the practitioner (Hinchliff et al., 2008). When applied well, nursing models explain how we, nurses, will complete the different stages of the nursing process (Aggleton and Chalmers, 2000) and provide an explanation for how the phenomenon which is nursing might work (Bender, 2017) (for more information on the nursing process, revisit Chapter 5). In addition, nursing models help to identify the appropriate assessment tools to use to help with the problem-solving process (for more on assessment tools, revisit Chapter 4). Linking the nursing model with the nursing process will enable you to assess, diagnose, plan, implement and evaluate structured, consistent and evidence-based nursing care where you critically examine the basis of your problem-solving and accurately and contemporaneously document the process (Peate, 2019). Remember that – in legal terms – if it is not documented, it did not happen. Completing Activity 7.2 will help you to identify some of the skills required of the practitioner for using a nursing model.

Activity 7.2   Critical thinking

What skills, including the 6Cs, do you think are required of the practitioner when using a nursing model?

An outline answer is given at the end of the chapter.

You might have thought about communication and assessment skills which require competence, but the skills required of the practitioner are more far-ranging than these. There are many nursing models available as nursing theorists think about how nursing activity can be appropriately articulated and framed. The nursing models in use are also being adapted and updated because of the dynamic nature of health and social care and the diversity of service users. This means that, as a nurse, you need to be aware of and understand a number of nursing models and when it is most appropriate to use a particular one. This will require not only knowledge of the models, but also the ability to quickly assess the nature of the problems individual patients present with in order to choose the right model to inform the more formal assessment process.

We will look at four of the main nursing models in use in this chapter. These are:

1. Roy's adaptation model;
2. Roper, Logan and Tierney's activities of daily living model;

3. Orem's self-care model; and

4. Neuman's system.

Each model will be followed by a case study to demonstrate application of the model to patient care.

Roy's adaptation model (Hinchliff et al., 2008)

The aim of this model is to help the patient develop coping strategies for different health statuses. These are:

*   physiological;
*   self-concept;
*   role functions; and
*   interdependence.

The assessment focuses on stimuli and stressors that underpin these in terms of the main cause of the problem, factors that can influence the problem and the beliefs and attitudes of the patient about the situation. Now read the following case study to see how the principles might be applied.

Case study: Enid's adjustment to the beginning of dementia

Enid was in her mid-seventies. She lived with her granddaughter, Imogen, and was very close to the family. Recently, she had started to forget things and was often found wandering in the street. Imogen took her to see the doctor. Enid was referred and seen by a consultant, who diagnosed her as living with dementia. Enid was devastated by this news, as was Imogen.

At home, the Admiral nurse, Ivy, talked through the diagnosis with Enid and Imogen. Because the diagnosis of dementia meant a lot of adjustments for Enid and Imogen, Ivy decided to use Roy's adaptation model to frame her assessment and care planning with Enid. Ivy asked Enid and Imogen to describe their daily life in order to identify potential triggers for Enid's change in behaviour. Ivy's assessment focused on:

*   how Enid thought about herself;
*   Enid's relationship with her granddaughter;
*   Enid's role in the family; and
*   any physical effects Enid was experiencing.

Ivy created a plan of care with Enid and Imogen that took into account their wishes and lifestyle. Ivy began by discussing their understanding of dementia. A short-term goal that Ivy identified was to increase their knowledge of dementia in order to give them confidence in

(Continued)

(Continued)

how to deal with it as well as what to expect going forward. Goal achievement would be evidenced if Enid and Imogen felt less anxious by the time they left the clinic. A longer-term goal was that Enid's relationship with her granddaughter was strengthened as her dependency increased. Therefore, Ivy recommended that Enid and Imogen talked about their shared history regularly and used photos to revisit significant events. Goal achievement would be evidenced by Enid being able to remember and engage with Imogen by talking about some past events. Ivy also suggested that Imogen tried to involve Enid in family activities. The goal here was to maintain and support Enid's role in the family for as long as possible.

In the case study above, you will have noted that Ivy's assessment of Enid has identified anxiety stemming from the medical diagnosis of early dementia. She has planned care that includes providing information about early dementia and ways of coping with it. It is important to recognise that even in short-term care environments such as an outpatient clinic, nurses still use nursing models to underpin their assessment and care planning with the patient. You can see how Roy's adaptation model (Hinchliff et al., 2008) is applied together with the nursing process in Figure 7.1, which shows the care plan for Enid in a format you might see used in practice.

Patient Name: Enid			
Patient Assessment	Nursing Diagnosis / Problem	Goals (SMART) / Strategy	Interventions / Implementation of Strategy
Self-Concept: Enid says she is anxious about her increasing forgetfulness, especially about her family history and relationships. Enid says she does not understand how dementia will affect her in the short and long term.	Enid is anxious about losing her identity and understanding of herself and her family history. Enid has little understanding of the potential impact of dementia on her life and relationships.	Short term: For Enid to be able to say she feels less anxious about her diagnosis. Long term: for Enid to develop and strengthen her relationship with Imogen while being able to continue to discuss their shared history. For Enid to be able to engage in family activities.	• Gain an understanding of what Enid and Imogen understand about dementia. • Provide verbal and written information about dementia to Enid and Imogen and identify other places they can access information and support: - Online. - Local support groups. - Day centre. • Provide support and reassurance and answer questions from Enid and Imogen and ask how they feel about things after getting some more information. • Prompt and encourage Imogen to talk with Enid about their shared family history; use photographs and other items to prompt memories. • Encourage Enid to be involved in things together with the family e.g. shopping, meals and gatherings.
Evaluation of Outcomes: On leaving the consultation, Enid and Imogen stated they felt more reassured about the future and understood a little more about living with dementia. They also took some literature and the details of a local day centre for people living with dementia. Enid and Imogen stated that they understood the value of reminiscing together and in continuing to ensure Enid is present and engaging in activities with the rest of the family. Enid said she was pleased about this as she felt she wanted to continue being 'gran' for as long as possible. They agreed to a follow up appointment in six months to review things.			

Figure 7.1 Enid's Care plan applying the Nursing Process and part of Roy's adaptation model

Completing Activity 7.3 will help you to identify other possible aspects that have not been mentioned in the case study.

Activity 7.3   Critical thinking

Read the case study about Enid again and consider the following questions:

- What other aspects of Enid's self-concept might you consider?
- What other aspects of Enid's relationship with her granddaughter might you want to think about?
- What physical aspects might also need to be considered?
- How is Ivy demonstrating using the 6Cs?

An outline answer is given at the end of the chapter.

We will now explore the use of Roper, Logan and Tierney's activities of daily living model.

Roper, Logan and Tierney's activities of daily living model (Roper et al., 2000)

The aim of this model is to consider factors that comprise daily living in a holistic and systematic way. The model takes account of 12 arenas that make up what are termed the *activities of daily living*:

1. maintaining a safe environment;
2. communicating;
3. breathing;
4. eating and drinking;
5. controlling body temperature;
6. washing and dressing;
7. working and playing;
8. mobilising;
9. eliminating;
10. expressing sexuality;
11. sleeping; and
12. dying.

The assessment focuses on all the areas and plans nursing interventions within those areas that are compromised, or potentially compromised. Now read the following case study to see how the principles might be applied.

Case study: Evan's trip to the seaside

You are on a learning disability placement, and this week the residents have a trip organised to go to the seaside. You are going with them and are responsible for Evan. Evan is a 14-year-old boy who has Down's syndrome. You check his care plan in order to identify what care you should be giving him. The care plan identifies that Evan requires some help with washing and dressing and that he occasionally becomes frustrated, leading to angry outbursts when in unfamiliar situations. He likes helping in the garden and enjoys art. You note that Evan does not appear to have any problems with eating and drinking or elimination. He is quite affectionate with people, which can sometimes be taken the wrong way.

You talk with Evan before the trip to find out how he feels about it and what he wants to do. Evan says that he wants to find some shells so that he can make a picture. He also wants to paddle in the sea. You ask Evan what he thinks the seaside will be like and who will be there. Evan says that he thinks there will be sand and water and shells. You tell Evan that there will be a lot of people there whom he will not know, and that it might be a good idea if he walks with you. You also suggest that he should tell you if he does not like something. You plan to bring drawing materials with you so that Evan can draw a picture of the seaside. You plan to use drawing as a distraction if Evan becomes agitated and frustrated, to try to avoid an outburst.

The trip to the seaside goes well. Evan wanted to give the waitress in the café a hug and you were able to explain that he was showing appreciation for the meal and the service. Evan did become frustrated when told that he had to leave the seaside. You suggested that he started to think about a picture of his day at the seaside on the way back to the bus and then gave him the drawing materials on the bus to complete the picture.

In the case study above, you will have noted the communication used to prepare Evan for his trip to the seaside. You will also have seen how a safe environment is maintained through suitable distraction techniques and supervision. This is shown in the extract from Evan's care plan, Figure 7.2, which shows how part of the model by Roper et al. (2000) is applied to Evan's care using the nursing process. Evan's expression of his sexuality in his affectionate approach to others is appropriately explained so that there is no offence taken.

Patient Name: Evan			
Patient Assessment	**Nursing Diagnosis / Problem**	**Goals (SMART) / Strategy**	**Interventions / Implementation of Strategy**
Maintaining a safe environment: Evan says he wants to play on the beach and find pebbles as well as paddle in the sea, but Evan is not always aware of what is safe and what is not.	Evan is not always able to express his needs to other people, such that other people may be alarmed by Evan's behaviour, which can include verbal and physical outbursts. Evan can become frustrated when asked to come away from a situation and struggles to manage his emotional response.	To help Evan to communicate his need to play and to keep Evan, and people around Evan, safe. To find other channels for Evan's energies so that he does not feel frustrated or anxious when he needs to leave a situation he is enjoying.	• Talk with Evan before the trip so that he can process what he wants from the trip and plan his activities. • Talk with Evan to understand his hope and aspirations for the trip and so that he understands he should tell staff when he wants to do something so they can keep him safe. • Talk with Evan about other things he likes to do which might help focus his attention should he start to feel frustrated or anxious. - Having discussed things with Evan, he wants to draw pictures of the seaside, so we will take drawing materials for him to use if he needs a distraction. • Talk with Evan about staying with staff to ensure he stays safe and that he understands the reasons for this. • Identify to Evan that he can say when he does not like a situation.
Evaluation of Outcomes: Evan was able to tell staff that he wanted to say thank you to a waitress who looked after him well and who was OK with having a hug when she understood this. Evan was unhappy when it was time to leave the beach but was able to quickly engage with his drawing materials on the bus and created a picture which showed what he had seen and done during the day. The distraction was positive for Evan as he enjoyed the drawing and was able to channel his energies into this. Evan says he was happy with the day and would not change anything about it.			

Figure 7.2 Evan's Care Plan applying the Nursing Process and part of Roper, Logan and Tierney's Activities of Daily Living Model

It is important to recognise that this model is suitable for use across a range of nursing contexts and settings. Completing Activity 7.4 will help you to consider the application of some of the other activities of daily living.

Activity 7.4 Critical thinking

Read the above case study again and consider the following questions:

- What other activities of daily living might be relevant here?
- What other aspects of maintaining a safe environment might need to be considered?
- In what way are the principles of the 6Cs demonstrated here?

An outline answer is given at the end of the chapter.

We will now explore the use of Orem's (2001) self-care model.

Orem's self-care deficit model (Orem, 2001)

This model recognises that people have capabilities and limitations for self-care as follows:

- self-care agency – relates to being able to take deliberate action to achieve desired goals (e.g. getting out of bed);
- universal self-care requisites – relates to what we need to take in in order to stay alive (e.g. fluid, food, air);
- developmental self-care requisites – relates to physical, functional and psychological development across the lifespan;
- health deviation self-care requisites – means how disorders can interfere with acquiring what is needed;
- helping methods and nursing systems – actions taken to help compensate or overcome limitations to patients' ability to act; and
- self-care deficit – something that individuals might do for themselves but for which they require help due to limitations in capabilities, such as cognitive, physical or psychological ability (e.g. deficits might be needing support with washing, moving about or decision-making).

The major assumption of Orem's model is that individuals should be self-reliant and responsible for their own care. On this basis, therefore, nursing action is required to support individuals in dealing with limitations to their ability to be self-caring; their self-care deficit. The therapeutic relationship we build with patients influences the assessment of their response as to whether they are managing or whether they need our help and support to attain the state where they are self-caring. Depending on the particular limitations an individual has, the nursing interventions required will be wholly compensatory (the nurse needs to do the whole of the intervention), partly compensatory (the nurse needs to do some of the intervention) or supportive-educative (the nurse needs to educate the person to self-care). Now read the following case study to see how the principles might be applied.

Case study: Patrick's rugby accident

Patrick sustained a shoulder injury that required surgery when playing rugby. His shoulder has been strapped following the surgery and he will be out of action for three months. Patrick, who is in his late twenties, is normally fit and well and will need to stay in hospital for a couple of days only. However, as his shoulder is strapped, he requires some help with washing and dressing and will not be able to carry things when he gets home. Sleeping is also awkward because he finds lying in bed painful.

Patrick is getting fed up with being reliant on other people to help him. His nurse, Margie, identifies that he has self-care deficits in that he will require nursing intervention to assist him with washing and dressing. He will also require pain relief and help with positioning at night to assist him to sleep. Margie shows him ways in which he can help himself with getting dressed. She also discusses with Patrick and his partner, Fern, how to continue when he is at home. By identifying what he can still do, Margie has helped ease some of Patrick's frustration, and he goes home in a better frame of mind to support his recovery and return to self-care.

In the above case study about Patrick, you may have noticed some of the helping roles that the nurse took in accordance with Orem's (2001) model. These include:

- partly compensatory, as the nurse assists with his washing and dressing but allows Patrick a role as well by guiding him to what he can do;
- wholly compensatory, by making sure he does not lift anything;
- educative – teaching him about the best position for sleeping and how to take his medication; and
- supporting him by offering psychological support to deal with his frustration.

Figure 7.3 shows how part of Orem's (2001) self-care deficit model is applied using the nursing process to a part of Patrick's care.

Patient Name: Patrick			
Patient Assessment	Nursing Diagnosis / Problem	Goals (SMART) / Strategy	Interventions / Implementation of Strategy
Self-care deficits: Patrick is frustrated with being unable to attend to his own washing and dressing needs as a result of the surgery to his shoulder.	Patrick has his shoulder strapped after surgery and is unable to wash and dress himself as a result of surgery.	To educate Patrick so that he can do as much washing and dressing for himself as possible as soon as possible. To support Patrick with the elements of washing and dressing he needs as he learns for himself how to do them in the short term. To educate Fern how to support Patrick with washing and dressing before Patrick is discharged home.	• Support Patrick to verbalise and overcome his frustrations about not being able to fully self-care at this time. • Identify with Patrick what he can do in the way of washing and dressing for himself. • Educate Patrick with some strategies to increase his ability to self-care with regard to washing and dressing. • Educate Fern with some strategies to help Patrick with regard to washing and dressing.
Evaluation of Outcomes: Patrick was able to talk about his frustration at not being able to wash and dress himself unaided. He was able to learn some strategies to help him address his deficits in this area after being shown ways in which he can help himself with washing and dressing. Fern was able to learn ways to support and enable Patrick to wash and dress without having to do everything for him.			

Figure 7.3 Patrick's Care Plan applying the Nursing Process and part of Orem's Self-Care Deficit Model

Completing Activity 7.5 will help you to consider other capabilities and limitations for self-care.

Activity 7.5   Critical thinking

Read the above case study again and consider the following questions:

- What other nursing systems could Margie use to help in her care planning for Patrick?
- What other limitations on self-care might also need to be considered?

An outline answer is given at the end of the chapter.

We now proceed to explore Neuman's system.

Neuman's system (Wilson et al., 2018)

This system is based on features that make us who we are, but which can also be variables that interact with each other in different ways depending on stress and personal factors. These are:

- physiological – relating to the anatomy and physiology of the person;
- psychological – relating to mental states, relationships and interaction with other people;
- sociocultural – with regard to background, beliefs and norms;
- developmental – relating to physical and psychological lifespan changes; and
- spiritual – with regard to belief systems.

Neuman sees health as a continuum of well-being that is constantly adapting to the environment (Wilson et al., 2018). Stressors arise from the internal and external environment and individual lines of resistance are used to try to mediate these threats. Now read the following case study to see how the principles might be applied.

Case study: Andrea's new baby

Andrea is 29 years old and has come into hospital to have her first baby. Her job is a nursing sister in a care home. Her husband, John, has recently been made redundant and her family live mostly abroad. She has a sister who lives 200 miles away. She started her maternity leave a month ago and was planning to take three months off work. However, John's redundancy means that she will have to go back to work as soon as possible.

Following the birth of her daughter, Andrea appears withdrawn and does not seem to be sleeping very well. The baby is well cared for and Andrea responds to her baby's needs appropriately. Kate, the midwife caring for Andrea, is concerned for her well-being. She wonders whether the stresses that Andrea has experienced with John losing his job and now the new baby bringing changes to their relationship will overwhelm Andrea's lines of resistance, which include her professional knowledge of healthcare and some family support (albeit at a distance). Kate decides to speak to Andrea about her situation and offer some advice and guidance. She will also check Andrea for postnatal depression and get her seen by a doctor as well.

It is clear from Kate's assessment of Andrea that she is developing depression. Kate talks to Andrea and John about what they can do to minimise the effects and build up Andrea's defences. She shows them some relaxation techniques. The doctor also prescribes medication to help Andrea.

Andrea goes home at the end of the week when her baby has regained her birth weight. Her sister comes to stay to help her out, and the community midwife and health visitor both check on the progress of both Andrea and her daughter. With this support in place, Andrea seems to be more able to cope. She continues on the medication for another month and seems more communicative and engaged with the people around her.

Completing Activity 7.6 will help you to consider other stressors and lines of resistance that may also be relevant when using this model.

Activity 7.6   Critical thinking

Read the above case study again and consider the following questions:

- What other stressors might Andrea have?
- What other lines of resistance (means of dealing with the stressors) are available to her?
- What else could Kate do?
- Which of the 6Cs is Kate using here?

You might like to try to create a partial care plan for Andrea along the lines of those done for Enid, Evan and Patrick, but this time using Neuman's system and the nursing process.

An outline answer is given at the end of the chapter.

We now proceed to looking at how a nursing model frames the assessment process.

How a nursing model frames the assessment process

Aggleton and Chalmers (2000) state:

The use of an appropriate nursing model informs assessment by establishing the kind of information required, the detail that is likely to be helpful and the ways in which the information might be best gathered.

(page 11)

The nursing model provides the conceptual framework from which activity flows. Dougherty et al. (2015) further identify:

Structuring patient assessment is vital to monitor the success of care and to detect the emergence of new problems. Nursing models provide frameworks for a systematic approach to assessment.

(page 10)

What this means is that if you are using a nursing model to frame the assessment process, it will ensure that you pay attention to relevant areas and are less likely to miss important cues. The models provide the structure for what might be holistic care planning; it is how you apply these with the patient that has the potential to make the assessment both holistic and person-centred. Table 7.1 sets out the different foci for assessment of the nursing models identified above.

Now read the following case study and complete Activity 7.7 in order to apply the different approaches to assessment relating to the different nursing models.

Case study: Bradley's development of epilepsy

Bradley is a mechanic. He is in his early twenties. After a night out with his mates six months ago, he was taken to hospital following a seizure. A number of tests were completed which showed that he had epilepsy. Bradley has found it difficult to come to terms with this diagnosis. He had to change his job because of not being able to drive, and now works for the council in the parks and gardens. The money is less, which is a worry for him. Three months ago, Bradley met a girl and they are becoming quite serious about each other. She is learning to cope with his fits. However, after another night out with his friends, he again is brought to accident and emergency with a longer seizure.

Activity 7.7   Critical thinking

Using the case study and Table 7.1, identify the main assessment points for Bradley when using the selected nursing models.

An outline answer is given at the end of the chapter.

Nursing model	Focus of assessment
Roy's adaptation model (Aggleton and Chalmers, 2000)	Adaptive problems (e.g. learning to live with a long-term condition).
	Patient experience (e.g. their narrative and description of how this is for them).
	Nursing diagnosis (e.g. anxiety about the developing relationship, not losing his girlfriend or job).
Roper, Logan and Tierney's activities of daily living model (Roper et al., 2000)	Biographical and health information such as the person's name, age, personal circumstances and reason for seeking health professional input.
	The person's ability to carry out the activities of daily living.
	Risk-assessing potential problems (e.g. personal injury during a fit).
Orem's self-care model (Orem, 2001)	Self-care capabilities: What resources and knowledge does the person have to be self-caring? What are the person's routines?
	Self-care limitations: What interferes with a person being able to self-care?
	Self-care agency: How has the person managed problems with being able to self-care?
Neuman's system (Wilson et al., 2018)	Person's perception of their situation: What are their health concerns?
	The effect of stressors on the person: How are things different?
	Your perception of the person and their situation: What do you see as the person's problem, and why?

Table 7.1   Foci for assessment with different nursing models

We now proceed to look at how nursing models also have an impact on decision-making in care planning (on decision-making in care planning, see also Chapter 9).

How a nursing model impacts on decision-making in care planning

As identified above, a nursing model directs the focus of assessment, and through this process also influences the decisions made for planning care. The transition from assessment to care planning involves critical thinking and clinical reasoning (Aston et al., 2010). Critical thinking means:

- evaluating assessment information; and
- forming judgements about the information you have.

When you are at the start of your nursing programme, you will probably follow the nursing model cues unquestioningly. However, as you develop knowledge and skill, you will start reasoning how applicable the model is for the patient's needs and consider the appropriate evidence to use for your care planning. Table 7.2 sets out the main considerations for decision-making in care planning for the nursing models identified above.

Nursing model	Focus of care planning
Roy's adaptation model (Aggleton and Chalmers, 2000)	The nursing diagnosis guides the care plan.
	Goals need to be short- and long-term.
	Nursing interventions are related to the stimulus for adaptation.
	Care planning should be evidence-based.
Roper, Logan and Tierney's activities of daily living model (Roper et al., 2000)	Helping people to return to independence.
	Teaching people what they need to know.
	Communicating information.
Orem's self-care model (Orem, 2001)	Prescribing nursing operations, which means the nursing interventions needed.
	Supporting self-care agency, which means involving individuals in their own care planning.
Neuman's system (Wilson et al., 2018)	Prioritising goals.
	Prevention as intervention, which means preventing someone either becoming unwell or becoming worse if already unwell.

Table 7.2 Care planning foci for different nursing models

Person-centredness and models of care

What we have seen is that models of care are tools for assessing and planning the care of patients on an individual, case-by-case basis. Some care providers try to create model care plans to be used with patients, but while these are useful in helping create understanding about a patient journey, e.g. through assessment, admission and after care related to surgery, they are not a replacement for person-centred assessment and care planning.

As we have seen in many of the activities and examples, people have different understandings of care and react to care environments in ways which are unique to them. Model care plans might identify some of the issues people in similar situations face, e.g. pain after surgery, but they cannot capture the individual's prior experiences of pain, their fear of pain, nor their individual response to pain relief, distraction and nursing support.

Models of care and the nursing process are therefore to be viewed as vital tools in the planning of care which is both holistic and person-centred. The ability to plan care in this way comes with practice and is premised on the ability to communicate effectively with people.

Activity 7.8   Decision-making

Read Bradley's case study again and now apply the different approaches to care planning when using the selected nursing models, as identified in Table 7.2.

An outline answer is given at the end of the chapter.

Conclusion

What has been highlighted is that the approaches stemming from the different nursing models focus on particular aspects of assessment and care decision-making. It is important that you are knowledgeable about a range of nursing models so that you can select the most appropriate model for your patient. Systematic assessment and care planning will ensure that you include and integrate all the relevant information from which to formulate the holistic care plan.

Systematic care planning means applying the model at the various stages of the nursing process. So each of the models' questions and assumptions needs to be accounted for in the assessment, diagnosis and planning of care.

Chapter summary

This chapter has identified the importance of understanding and selecting from a range of nursing models to reflect different approaches to care in a variety of settings. These models are important for articulating nursing activity and the values and beliefs that underpin nursing. Summarising application of some of the principles associated with selected nursing models through the case studies supplied and the activities has given you the opportunity to think critically about how you might use nursing models in practice.

Activities: brief outline answers

Activity 7.1   Reflection (page 113)

You might have identified Roper, Logan and Tierney's activities of daily living model, Orem's self-care model, Roy's adaptation model and Neuman's system as nursing models you have seen used in placements. You may have identified that a particular nursing model reflected the type and level of support required by the patients in that area. You might also have considered how the model changed the focus of your assessment questioning in terms of whether the patient was returning to self-caring or adapting to a different health status. If there was no nursing model in evidence, you might have found yourself having to describe your assessment and care planning 'blind', and therefore potentially from a task-based perspective rather than underpinned by sound nursing principles.

Activity 7.2   Critical thinking (page 114)

The skills required of the practitioner are:

- observation skills;
- communication skills;
- decision-making skills;
- assessment skills;
- nursing diagnostic skills for making a nursing diagnosis; and
- critical thinking skills.

Communication and Competence, as in being able to apply the model, are the 'Cs' from the 6Cs in use here.

Activity 7.3   Critical thinking (page 117)

Other aspects of Enid's self-concept that you might have considered are:

- not knowing who she is anymore;
- lack of confidence in herself;
- fear of the future; and
- viewing herself as less capable.

Other aspects of Enid's changing relationship with her granddaughter, Imogen, which you might have considered are:

- switching of roles as Enid's dependency increases;
- more stressors on the relationship; and
- the illness overtaking Enid's identity as a grandmother.

Physical aspects that might need to be considered include:

- Deterioration in Enid's short-term memory, which might create safety concerns such as forgetting to turn the oven off, or checking the temperature of food or drink before ingesting or water before bathing.
- Other issues may emerge, such as issues with mobility, eating and drinking, and continence management.

Ivy is demonstrating using compassion by allowing Enid and Imogen time to adjust and by working with what is familiar to them, and is doing so in a caring manner. Commitment is demonstrated by looking at longer-term goals. Communication is used through the different strategies offered and the holistic nature of the assessment demonstrates that she is competent at what she is doing.

Activity 7.4   Critical thinking (page 119)

Other activities of daily living that you might have considered are:

- washing and dressing if Evan spilt something on himself or was sick;
- working and playing as Evan likes to make pictures as part of the way in which he relaxes; and
- elimination in terms of how this would be supervised; to use a public toilet for example.

Other aspects of maintaining a safe environment include what you would do if Evan did have an angry outburst and how you would manage this. You would need to consider:

- Evan's safety, making sure that he could not harm himself;
- the safety of others, making sure that they were able to remove themselves from potential harm; and
- your safety.

The 6Cs are demonstrated through the communication used, the care strategies considered and used to demonstrate some competence, and courage is shown in arranging the trip.

Activity 7.5   Critical thinking (page 122)

Other nursing systems that Margie might have considered include:

- taking a nursing history about patterns of living; and
- using pain assessment tools.

As regards limitations on self-care, Patrick may not be able to cut up food and may also require advice with sexual needs.

Activity 7.6   Critical thinking (page 123)

Other stressors for Andrea might be:

- not wanting people to know that she has professional knowledge because it does not relate to children;
- worrying that people expect her to know what to do;
- trying to manage her relationship with her husband at the same time as developing a relationship with her child;
- money worries; and
- returning to work so soon.

Other lines of resistance that Andrea could draw on might be:

- her professional knowledge of caring for others;
- a shared history with her husband;
- continuing more frequent contact with her sister;
- drawing on the experience of work colleagues; and
- talking to the mortgage lender and seeking financial advice.

Other areas that Kate could also consider include:

• referring Andrea to a counsellor and to self-help groups.

Kate is using the 6Cs through showing her commitment and compassion for Andrea by recognising how she is feeling and communicating with her and her husband to identify the resources she has. She is also showing her competence in being able to identify these with Andrea.

Activity 7.7   Critical thinking (page 125)

When using Roy's adaptation model, your assessment is likely to have focused on Bradley's ability to adjust to having epilepsy and still remain within his circle of friends. Your nursing diagnosis might have been around anxiety relating to knowledge of the condition as well as interpersonal and economic factors.

When using Roper, Logan and Tierney's activities of daily living model, your assessment is likely to have focused on maintaining a safe environment by assessing Bradley's vital signs and consciousness and considering his ability to carry on working safely. You might also have risk-assessed the potential for Bradley to injure himself while having a fit, and for him to develop depression because of not yet having come to terms with his condition.

When using Orem's self-care deficit model, your assessment is likely to have focused on Bradley's ability to take care of himself physically given his lifestyle and the unpredictability of the seizures. You might have identified that he requires nursing support in providing information for him and his girlfriend on ways they can take control of his care.

When using Neuman's system, your assessment is likely to have focused on whether Bradley feels stressed and what his main stressor is – is it that he worries about losing this job or his girlfriend leaving? You would think about discussing this with Bradley to find out how he is feeling and what his perception is. You would also ask how he normally manages his epilepsy and how he wants to be involved in his care. Your perception of Bradley's problem is likely to be that he is a young man in denial of his condition and in a serious relationship that is important to him.

Activity 7.8   Decision-making (page 127)

When using Roy's adaptation model, your care planning is likely to focus on the nursing diagnosis that Bradley lacks insight into his condition and that he is anxious. The short-term goal that you may consider for Bradley is that he will be fully informed about his condition and treatment within one week. The longer-term goal that you may have identified is that Bradley is less anxious by the end of one month. Your care plan may include stress alleviation strategies such as talking, relaxation techniques and identifying where to get further support (e.g. financial benefits).

When using Roper, Logan and Tierney's activities of daily living model, your care plan is likely to focus on communicating information about Bradley's condition and treatment and interpreting this, as appropriate. You might also have considered the nursing observations required, such as neurological observations and positioning Bradley to ensure his breathing is supported. It is likely that you will also have considered teaching Bradley about his medication regimen.

When using Orem's self-care model, your care plan is likely to focus on prescribing the nursing interventions required, including educative components, compensatory strategies and support. These are likely to have included informing Bradley about why his seizures follow his nights out and what he can do about this. It is likely that you will involve Bradley in his washing and dressing and talk to him about ways of reducing his anxiety and stress.

When using Neuman's system, your care planning is likely to focus on prioritising Bradley's recovery from the seizure and ensuring medication is given on time. You would then consider how to reduce his anxiety and stress to prevent more seizures. You would also need to plan how to help him gain some control through providing information.

Further reading

Aston, L, Wakefield, J and McGown, R (eds) (2010) *The Student Nurse Guide to Decision Making in Practice*. Maidenhead: Open University Press.

This book is useful for outlining the decision-making skills required of the developing nurse and how to make use of evidence and team members to determine a course of action.

Hall, C and Ritchie, D (2013) *What Is Nursing? Exploring Theory and Practice* (3rd edn). London: SAGE.

An introduction to the world of nursing, incorporating views from student and qualified nurses.

Holland, K and Jenkins, J (2019) *Applying the Roper, Logan and Tierney Model in Practice* (3rd edn). London: Churchill Livingstone.

A book which explores the use of the Roper model using the activities of daily living.

Hinchliff, S, Norman, S and Schober, J (eds) (2008) *Nursing Practice and Health Care* (5th edn). London: Hodder Arnold.

This book identifies some of the different nursing models, giving examples of their use.

Useful websites

www.currentnursing.com/nursing_theory/

A good overview of a number of nursing theories.

www.nursing-theory.org/theories-and-models/

A very brief overview of a number of nursing models and theories.

Chapter 8 Ethical aspects of patient assessment

Peter Ellis

NMC Future Nurse: Standards of Proficiency for Registered Nurses

This chapter will address the following platforms and proficiencies:

Platform 1: Being an accountable professional

At the point of registration, the registered nurse will be able to:

1.1   understand and act in accordance with *The Code: Professional standards of practice and behaviour for nurses, midwives and nursing associates*, and fulfil all registration requirements.

1.2   understand and apply relevant legal, regulatory and governance requirements, policies, and ethical frameworks, including any mandatory reporting duties, to all areas of practice, differentiating where appropriate between the devolved legislatures of the United Kingdom.

1.9   understand the need to base all decisions regarding care and interventions on people's needs and preferences, recognising and addressing any personal and external factors that may unduly influence their decisions.

1.14 provide and promote non-discriminatory, person-centred and sensitive care at all times, reflecting on people's values and beliefs, diverse backgrounds, cultural characteristics, language requirements, needs and preferences, taking account of any need for adjustments.

1.19 act as an ambassador, upholding the reputation of their profession and promoting public confidence in nursing, health and care services.

Platform 3: Assessing needs and planning care

At the point of registration, the registered nurse will be able to:

3.15 demonstrate the ability to work in partnership with people, families and carers to continuously monitor, evaluate and reassess the effectiveness of all agreed nursing plans and care, sharing decision making and readjusting agreed goals, documenting progress and decisions made.

3.16   demonstrate knowledge of when and how to refer people safely to other professionals or services for clinical intervention or support.

Platform 4: Providing and evaluating care

At the point of registration, the registered nurse will be able to:

4.1   demonstrate and apply an understanding of what is important to people and how to use this knowledge to ensure their needs for safety, dignity, privacy, comfort and sleep can be met, acting as a role model for others in providing evidence-based person-centred care.
4.2   work in partnership with people to encourage shared decision making in order to support individuals, their families and carers to manage their own care when appropriate.
4.3   demonstrate the knowledge, communication and relationship management skills required to provide people, families and carers with accurate information that meets their needs before, during and after a range of interventions.

Chapter aims

After reading this chapter, you will be able to:

- understand the relevance of ethical theories to patient assessment and care planning;
- relate ethical principles, including autonomy, beneficence, non-maleficence and justice, to patient assessment;
- discuss the nature of best interests and how these might contribute to the patient care planning process;
- identify some problems with ethics as theory and ethics in practice; and
- begin to problem-solve ethical difficulties in patient assessment and resource allocation.

Introduction

Case study: Nancy's ethical dilemma

Nancy is working in a mental health day unit where a number of the older patients who attend have early dementia. One woman, Sybil, has been coming for a number of months and Nancy has built a close therapeutic relationship with her. Sybil lives with her daughter, Gloria. Gloria works part-time on the days that Sybil is at the day unit. Sybil has recently been complaining to Nancy that her daughter is locking her in her bedroom and hiding

(Continued)

(Continued)

her money. She says she has been asking her grandson, Luke, for money and he has given her some of his pocket money. She says she has been asking Luke to run errands for her such as posting her replies to begging letters. Nancy is concerned about this. She considers whether she can break Sybil's confidentiality and speak to Gloria about this as she is concerned about Sybil's vulnerability to scams and the involvement of her grandson.

Ethics underpin healthcare practice and are written into *The Code: Professional standards of practice and behaviour for nurses, midwives and nursing associates* (NMC, 2018b) with clear expectations of how practitioners are expected to conduct themselves. The above case study raises ethical issues in relation to confidentiality, autonomy and mental capacity. It also raises the spectre of financial abuse, which is a serious safeguarding issue (Social Care Institute for Excellence, 2020). This chapter will introduce some of the main ethical theories that inform health and social care practice. It will identify how these relate to patient assessment and care planning. You will be given the opportunity to explore ethical problems relating to patient assessment and care planning after you have had the chance to learn more about ethical principles, and will be asked to return to Nancy's case study above to discuss the dilemma described in Activity 8.4. The chapter will also ask you to consider issues about translating ethical theory into practice.

Ethical theories

Morality and ethics are key underpinnings for the actions that health and social care professionals take (Ellis, 2020). Ethical and moral decision-making in any walk of life is best guided by the use of ethical theory and the ethical principles which underlie these. As with using models of nursing to guide patient assessment, ethical theory gives structure to ethical decision-making and guides the user towards making a decision that is based on ethical reasoning. The two main ethical theories that are cited in healthcare ethics texts are *consequentialism* and *deontology*; although these are by no means the only theories that can be used. We will look at these two theories in more detail now.

Simply put, consequentialism considers that the consequences of an action may be used to justify an action that has been taken (Ellis, 2019). That is, the ends justify the means; if the results of the action the healthcare professionals take benefit the person, then this justifies whatever actions are taken to reach that goal. The *benefit* is hard to define, but classic utilitarians would say an action is justified if it achieved the greatest benefit (happiness) for the most people. For example, when a new drug becomes available, organisations such as the National Institute for Health and Care Excellence will not only consider its efficacy, but also the ethics of distribution in terms of how the greatest number of people can benefit within economic constraints. So, if the action is spending money on an expensive drug, how many people will it benefit, and by how much, compared to spending the same amount of money on a less expensive drug, or indeed not spending the money at all? Read the case study below to help you understand this theory.

Case study: Keeping a secret

Pearl is a resident in a care home in which you are on placement. Pearl has been living with dementia for many years and now has very little in the way of short-term memory. Pearl has been in the home for several years and is well known to the staff. Pearl's husband, Ken, used to visit her several times a week but he has recently died. Pearl attended Ken's funeral but has no memory of going. Pearl often asks the staff where Ken is and becomes upset when they tell her he is dead. One member of the team who knows Pearl well, Loretta, suggests that perhaps people should tell Pearl he is coming later rather than that he is dead. Some of the team are uncomfortable with lying, but Pearl seems happy with the explanation, which is repeated to her several times a day.

Activity 8.1 Critical thinking

Is lying in this instance a reasonable thing to do? Explain your answer.

An outline answer is given at the end of the chapter.

Deontology

Deontology considers the motivation behind actions and whether these are morally just. This is determined by rules and obligations of duty such as are embedded in *The Code*. Deontology is reflective of the Judaeo-Christian tradition of following one's duties and 'doing as you would be done by'. Deontologists are also sometimes called 'rule-based theorists' because they always follow the rules no matter what situation they find themselves in. For example, no matter how busy the placement area is, if a patient has been incontinent, they would expect you to help clean them up and not leave them wet. Read the following case study to help you understand this theory.

Case study: Rohan's first shift in accident and emergency

Rohan was on his third placement in an accident and emergency department. A prisoner called Bruce was brought in with a broken arm following an assault in prison. Rohan was asked by his practice supervisor Claire to assist in plastering Bruce's arm.

Claire asked one of the accompanying prison officers, Tony, what had happened to Bruce. Tony replied that Bruce was in prison for rape, and therefore a target for other prisoners. They had cornered him during lunch and broken his arm by snapping it across a table.

(Continued)

(Continued)

Rohan was surprised at how calmly Claire took this news and that she spoke kindly to Bruce as she plastered his arm, checking he was not in any undue pain. At the end of the procedure, Claire explained the plaster observations to Bruce, the prison officers and Rohan. Bruce thanked her and was escorted back to the prison van. Rohan found this all rather difficult to take in.

Activity 8.2 Reflection

In Chapter 2, you were asked to reflect on situations where you might find it difficult to provide unbiased care. Now put yourself in Rohan's situation and think about how you might react. What do you need to consider in order to give professional and unbiased care?

Although this activity is based on your experience, there is a limited outline answer at the end of the chapter.

Among the most widely cited of the principles that guide modern ethical thinking are those identified by Beauchamp and Childress (2013), which are *beneficence, non-maleficence, autonomy* and *justice*. These principles guide actions through identifying what our duty might be in a given situation and are therefore part of the deontological tradition. It is worth understanding each of these principles as they play an important role in modern ethical thinking.

Beneficence

Beneficence means *doing good* for the person. For example, health promotion aims to improve the health of individuals by helping them to help themselves. Such an activity would be classed as doing good. In this sense, *doing good* has quite a broad definition, and not only means giving good nursing care, but also refers to the manner in which the care is delivered, treating people well and with respect.

Non-maleficence

Non-maleficence means not doing harm. Risk assessment is a fundamental part of healthcare practices in order to avoid doing harm to patients. It is unlikely that a healthcare practitioner would deliberately set out to do harm to the person in their care (although, sadly, there have been some exceptions). It is incumbent on health and social care professionals and considered good practice to incorporate risk assessment within the assessment and care planning process in order to ensure that plans are in place to avoid doing harm (to look again at how this can be done, revisit Chapters 6 and 7).

That said, this principle can never be taken too literally in health and social care because a lot of the things we do actually cause some harm in order to benefit the person in the long term (e.g. vaccination, which initially hurts – causes harm – but has a benefit to the person in the long term). The principle of not doing harm really means do not do deliberate harm, or if you inflict some harm ensure it is in the process of doing some good and that the doing good is your intention.

Autonomy

Autonomy recognises that individuals have the right to make their own decisions. For example, it is up to individuals when they want to get washed or dressed or when they want to go to bed, rather than having to fit in with a health and social care routine. Equally, while it may be considered in patients' interests to stop drinking alcohol or reduce their weight or modify their diet, it is nevertheless their autonomous right to choose whether or not to do so. We will discuss best interests, both as an ethical concept and as they apply in UK law, at the end of the chapter.

Justice

Justice is about the shared benefits and burdens of society, about treating everyone fairly (Ellis, 2020). It might also be considered that it is a contract between people whereby if that person has given what is asked, they can expect something in return. Health and social care is both a benefit and a burden to society as a whole in terms of receiving care and finding the money to resource that care. Justice requires that people with the same or broadly similar needs are essentially treated the same regardless of anything else. As the code of professional standards of practice and behaviour for nurses, midwives and nursing associates requires, act with honesty and integrity at all times, treating people fairly and without discrimination, bullying or harassment (NMC, 2018b).

We now proceed to consider the relevance of ethical theories for patient assessment and care planning.

The relevance of ethical theories for patient assessment and care planning

Ethical theories inform the philosophies of care that guide health and social care practice and for which practitioners are held accountable by service users (Lloyd, 2010). A philosophy of care is a statement about the values and beliefs that inform practice within a given area. It is these values and beliefs that are said to inform the ways in which care is delivered and how staff behave. The moral principles of autonomy, beneficence, non-maleficence and justice have implications for patient assessment and care planning in a number of ways, particularly where the values and behaviours of the 6Cs have not been observed. The values and behaviours of the 6Cs are about demonstrating care and compassion through recognising a person's autonomy and dignity of being. We will now consider how the four principles might apply to the process of care planning.

Autonomy

Autonomy assumes that patients have a right to be involved, or perhaps even take the leading role, in decisions about their care. Within assessment, it is important to gather relevant data without trying to control what the person says or reveals, and to do so in a non-judgemental manner, because people have the right to lead their lives as they choose (so long as it does not interfere with the rights of others).

Following on from assessing, when planning care, health and social care professionals may make recommendations, but it is up to individuals whether they take these up or not. The Mental Capacity Act 2005 is quite clear that people should be assumed to have capacity to make decisions unless it has been proven that they have not. The Act is also clear that people with capacity have the right to make decisions with which others may disagree, so in planning care with an individual who has capacity, and can therefore exercise autonomy, the plan made needs to reflect what they have decided. In cases where a person lacks capacity, and therefore is unable to exercise autonomy, any decisions about their care need to reflect what they might have chosen when they had capacity and be in their best interests. Reading the case study below may help you to make more sense of this.

Case study: William's deteriorating health

William is a 72-year-old retired railway worker who lives with his wife, Marjorie, in a bungalow. Marjorie has noticed that William appears to be becoming more confused. He forgets where he has put things and important dates, and she often finds him wandering around the house in the night. William had a fall and sustained a sprained ankle. He is admitted to the medical assessment unit. Marjorie insists that William cannot do anything for himself and proceeds to tell you that you need to tell him what to do. Marjorie constantly tells William what to do, and William appears agitated and confused and says that he wants to go and meet his friends for a pint.

You make Marjorie a cup of tea and ask her to wait outside while you undertake your assessment of William. William is not able to answer a number of your assessment questions and repeatedly says he needs to go. You identify that he has memory problems and therefore is not sure where he is. You tell him where he is on a number of occasions and reinforce this information as required.

You identify that William is capable of expressing a preference for what he likes to eat or drink and whether he wants you to touch his ankle. William is also able to tell you whether he is in pain or not. However, you do have concerns about his ability to make decisions about his care arrangements, especially when he is discharged, and you communicate these concerns to the healthcare team.

Activity 8.3   Critical thinking

The case study above identifies some problems about William being able to make his own decisions. Consider the following questions:

- How is William's autonomy affected?
- What does the Mental Capacity Act 2005 have to say about this?
- What else might you need to consider?
- How does this relate to the principles of the 6Cs?

An outline answer is given at the end of the chapter.

Beneficence

Beneficence, as identified earlier, relates to doing good. With this focus in mind, you need to ensure your assessment considers the welfare of the patient and that at all times you are promoting their health and well-being. Taken alongside autonomy, doing good for the patient also means that you empower the patient to identify what good means to them (i.e. the patient is the person who defines what the proposed outcomes of care are). Read the following case study to help you to understand how this might translate into practice.

Case study: Henry's reluctance to engage

Henry is an 81-year-old man who lives with his daughter, Miranda. He has had incontinence issues for some time now and has become more and more reclusive, withdrawing from family interaction and engagement with people in general. The community continence nurse has been to visit him and explained options available to help him manage his incontinence. However, Henry would rather continue using a bottle, which he misses a lot of the time, thereby wetting his clothing and his bed sheets, which Miranda has to deal with every day. Miranda is at her wits' end and finds Henry's stubbornness very unhelpful.

(Continued)

(Continued)

Henry has a son, Graham, who lives in the next county. Graham has invited Henry to come and stay so that Miranda gets a break. Henry is concerned about going because of his incontinence problems and refuses to visit Graham. Miranda talks to the community nursing team and asks them if there is anything they can do. The community nurse, Jill, gets in touch with the continence nurse again and arranges a meeting with Henry. They discuss the urisheath system, which will enable Henry to travel while being incontinent and might make his life easier when he stays with Graham.

Henry is at first reluctant, but as Graham and his wife have a baby daughter, Henry is keen to spend time with his new granddaughter and finally agrees to try the new device and go to visit his son. Jill is careful to explain tactfully how to fit the urisheath and how to manage it and allows Henry time to get used to the idea. She leaves the urisheath for Henry to examine in his own time in private. She visits a few times to help Henry become more expert in using it.

Henry visited Graham and enjoyed spending time with his new granddaughter. He is continuing to use the urisheath and is now able to engage better with Miranda and her family.

The case study above highlights the need for patient assessment specifically to identify problems and plan solutions that not only have a healthcare benefit, but which also promote patient well-being and autonomy. Health and social care recommendations may not always be welcomed immediately, but when care planning is shared and the benefits, *the good*, for patients are communicated and clarified in such a way that they can understand, then patients are more likely to see how proposed interventions can help them.

Non-maleficence

Non-maleficence is about not doing harm, as identified earlier. This can also be related to the competence element of the 6Cs. From this perspective, the assessment focuses on risk-assessing actual and potential problems. Care planning follows this with nursing interventions to prevent such problems occurring, or to minimise their impact. Read the following case study to help you understand this better in terms of patient assessment and care planning.

Case study: Eve's diabetic foot

Eve is 65 years old and has been living with diabetes for the last five years. She has now been prescribed insulin and is finding this very cumbersome because it interrupts her day. Eve normally enjoys going on walking holidays and visiting art galleries, but unfortunately she has started to develop neuropathy as her lack of blood sugar control has damaged the nerve endings in her feet, which makes walking difficult.

Eleanor is a student nurse on a community placement with the practice nurse, who Eve comes to see for her regular check-up. Eleanor notices that Finola, the practice nurse, pays special attention to Eve's feet and examines them closely. Eleanor also notices that the skin is discoloured and dry and that Eve's toenails look gnarled and a different colour. Finola gives Eve advice on how to look after her feet, especially the skin. She refers Eve to the podiatrist for specialist help with her toenails.

When Eve has gone, Eleanor asks Finola why she did not offer to cut Eve's toenails, as they looked rather long. Finola explains that because Eve is a diabetic, there are risks attached to cutting toenails, such as introducing infection through a sharp nail scratching a neighbouring toe, or a nick of the skin; people with diabetes should therefore have podiatric assistance with foot care. Finola emphasises that care planning includes risk-assessing potential problems such as infection and planning how to avoid these potential harms. Eleanor now appreciates the importance of including potential problems in care planning processes.

The case study above highlights the importance of risk-assessing potential harm that patients may do themselves as well as any potential harm that may result from health professionals not giving necessary information. Care planning to safeguard the patient may also need to involve other members of the health and social care team.

Justice

Justice within patient assessment and care planning relates to the equitable distribution of nursing interventions, resources and time. Read the following case study to understand how this might relate to practice.

Case study: Zoe's sheet dilemma

It was Christmas on the stroke ward and, due to norovirus, many staff were off sick and some of the patients were affected too. Consequently, the ward was short-staffed. Zoe, the nurse in charge, needed to prioritise to ensure the patients received the care they needed. She was on shift with only two other staff – one qualified and one healthcare assistant. Between them, they determined who had the priority needs and explained to the patients why they might not be immediately available to provide care. Many of the patients had been incontinent or sick and needed changing. As it was Christmas, the ward was short of sheets and none were available from other wards. Zoe made the decision to change all the bottom sheets that were wet and replace these with the top sheet and provide blankets or duvets instead for covering the patients. Those who had also been sick received the last clean sheets available. Although not an ideal solution, it nevertheless meant that all the patients were left clean and comfortable.

The case study above highlights a very real situation where nurses frequently have to problem-solve. Ethical ideas of justice would expect that all the patients with wet beds would be treated equally and receive clean sheets. However, as this case study has demonstrated, equality is not always possible within finite resources, and therefore clinical judgement has to play a part. Patient assessment is crucial to this for identifying priorities as well as risk-assessing the potential for harm. This highlights that translating ethics into practice can sometimes be problematic. We now proceed to explore some such problems.

Problems with ethics as theory and ethics in practice

Problems with ethics as theory and ethics in practice often relate to resourcing issues. For example, waiting lists are the result of many people requiring treatment but there being limited spaces available or staff to provide the treatments people are waiting for. Equally, problems may arise from a mismatch in ethical thinking and ethical behaviour. For example, you may talk about non-discriminatory practice but may have identified that you do need to discriminate in order to provide necessary care. Aston et al. (2010) make the point that 'in everyday practice there are often situations where it can be difficult to know whether we are truly acting in the patient's best interests' (page 90). This is especially true where patients come from different cultures and where you may find it difficult to integrate different world views. Consider the following case study, which may help your understanding.

Case study: Biji's sexual assault

Biji is a 20-year-old student studying law at university. She is admitted to the gynaecology ward with vaginal injuries after she was raped on the way home from a party. Biji is a Hindu and does not want her family to know because of the shame this would bring on them. She is clearly distressed and in need of support. You find it hard to understand how this assault could be viewed as her fault by her family. You talk it over with Biji, but she is adamant that she does not want her family to know.

Her mother visits that afternoon and asks you what is wrong with Biji. Because Biji has expressly forbidden you telling her family, you say that that information is confidential, and she will have to ask Biji herself. Later you see Biji and her mother arguing, and when her mother leaves Biji is in floods of tears. You go to comfort her but she is inconsolable because her mother has disowned her. You try to reassure Biji that her mother will come round but she says that you do not understand her culture.

You are not sure what to do next, so you go to speak to your practice supervisor about this. Your practice supervisor identifies that you did the right thing by not breaking Biji's confidentiality and allowing her to make the decision herself about what she told her mother. Nevertheless, it would have been helpful to have had a member of staff there for additional support for Biji when she spoke to her mother. Your practice supervisor advises that you inform yourself about different religious and cultural rules and practices in order to be better prepared in the future.

Biji's case study highlights how differences in world views can sometimes constrain communication and the therapeutic relationship. Although Biji's confidentiality has not been broken, ethical questions nevertheless remain about whether this has resulted in doing her good and not doing her harm. Equally, the 6Cs highlight that care should also be compassionate, that health professionals should show commitment to patient need and use courage in approaching patients' problems. Moral dilemmas result from the fact that choices need to be made from different alternatives and it may be difficult to predict the consequences of decision-making in practice. For example, a treatment list may need to be cancelled or curtailed and it will be clinicians who decide who is prioritised for treatment. This impinges on the autonomy of individuals to make decisions for themselves, but may in fact be a fair exercise of justice. Aston et al. (2010) suggest that we need to consider how good, right, fair, honest and empowering our decision-making is when faced with such ethical dilemmas.

Nurses are morally accountable to do their best for patients (Wilkinson, 2016). In fact, *The Code* requires nurses to 'put the interests of people using or needing nursing or midwifery services first' (NMC, 2018b, page 6). In terms of care planning, this means accepting responsibility to give good care that is effective, legal and competent. As a student, you may feel that you are not always competent to do what is asked of you. It is therefore important that you make known to your practice supervisor, or other team member, that you do not feel proficient to carry out the task, and then follow this up by extending your knowledge. The same applies if a patient asks you to do something that you are not sure about.

Maintaining confidentiality is an area that has been problematic and difficult in ethical terms. Revisit the case study about Nancy's ethical dilemma at the start of the chapter. When you have read the case study again, complete Activity 8.4 in order to problem-solve some of the ethical issues.

Activity 8.4   Critical thinking

You will have identified some concerns within the case study of Nancy's ethical dilemma. Make a list of what you see as the ethical issues arising in this case. Now answer the following questions:

- What does Nancy need to consider?
- What can Nancy do?
- Who else might Nancy involve?

An outline answer is given at the end of the chapter.

Best interests

It is worthwhile stopping for a moment before concluding this chapter about ethical aspects to consider the idea of best interests in more detail. As we have seen at various points in this chapter, care planning for patients needs to account for whatever is in the best interests of the patient, but what best interests are all about is not always that easy to understand. For example, what does 'best interests' mean? Who defines 'best interests'? And who decides what is in someone's best interests when they cannot decide for themselves?

These questions are growing in importance as the population ages and diseases such as dementias become increasingly prevalent. Best interests decisions are widely seen in care planning used by carers and nurses working in social care and are used as the justification for plans of care and care delivery to people who are not themselves able to participate in the care planning process.

We also saw in Biji's case that the nurse might have considered it to be in Biji's best interests to discuss what had happened with her family, because in the nursing view the support the family might offer is seen as valuable. We saw on the other hand that, from a cultural viewpoint, discussing the rape is not something that people from some cultures do, so might not work in Biji's best interests. This gives us an idea of what is meant by best interests.

On the one hand there are interests that people have which might be termed physical; Benjamin and Curtis (2010) refer to decision-making, which is focussed on physical interests as making medical decisions in the *technical sense.*

Other decision-making is less objective and might refer to the culture and context within which the person lives. Examples of this are referred to by Benjamin and Curtis

(2010) as medical decisions in the contextual sense. It is through communication and understanding that nurses can assess and plan care which responds to the contextual, person-centred needs of the patient.

Such context is often given by family and members of the multidisciplinary team who know, or have known, the patient for some time – perhaps even when they still had capacity. Other sources of information for nurses undertaking care planning for people who may no longer be able to express what they regard as being in their best interests include paying attention to records of previously expressed wishes, such as advance care plans and advance statements.

The need to identify and care plan in the best interests of people is also tied up with UK law in the form of the Mental Capacity Act 2005, which states: 'An act done, or decision made, under this Act for or on behalf of a person who lacks capacity must be done, or made, in his best interests'. These decisions 'must consider, so far as is reasonably ascertainable … the person's past and present wishes and feelings (and, in particular, any relevant written statement made by him when he had capacity'.

Understanding best interests and what they mean therefore provides the nurse with a good understanding of the nature of person-centred care planning and why it is desirable from a nursing and ethical point of view. Best interests and person-centred care planning are in this sense inextricably linked.

Case study: Planning Michael's care

Michael is a newly admitted resident in a nursing home. Michael has advanced vascular dementia and does not know where he is, does not recognise his family, or who the care staff are or what they do. Michael can get very angry at times and was becoming physical with his family, although as he is elderly and also has arthritis, this is not as much of a problem as it once was, but it is enough of an issue for them to seek his admission to the home.

Bella, a nurse, is tasked with writing Michael's care plan, but has very little to go on as Michael was cared for at home by his family prior to the admission. Bella is an experienced nursing home nurse and takes Sui Minh, a student, to one side to discuss how they might assess Michael's needs. Sui Minh thinks they will be able to work his needs out from his diagnosis and Bella's experience, but Bella says there is more to it than that.

Bella suggests they have a conversation with Michael's social worker and get a copy of his social care plan, which will have some of his information on it. Through this they identify that Michael had also attended a day centre until recently, so they are able to talk to the staff there and get an insight into the sort of things Michael liked doing, such as listening to jazz music.

(Continued)

(Continued)

Bella also suggests they make an appointment with the family in order to discuss Michael's social history, such as places he had been and the work he had done as well as understanding what had worked in the way of care for him when he was living at home. Sui Minh was surprised at how much information they were able to gather about Michael, and the way in which Bella was able to use this to create plans for care, including strategies for keeping Michael calm and reacting to episodes when he was upset.

What Sui Minh is seeing, although she may not be aware of it, is Bella attempting to create a care plan which represents Michael's best interests. She does this by understanding the things that are important to him as a person rather than concentrating on his medical diagnosis. The information Bella collects from family and friends and people who know Michael is about the context of Michael's life and so represent what we identified earlier as medical decisions in the contextual sense – that is care planning for Michael which is about who he is and has been, rather than about the disease he now lives with.

Activity 8.5 Reflection

Consider the last occasion when you undertook a care plan assessment. Make a list of the places you gathered information about the patient you were care planning for. Think about the various sources of information and what they contributed to the care planning process. Where else might you have got information and what might this have added to the process?

As this activity is based on your experience, there is no outline answer at the end of the chapter.

What you might have identified is that you used very few sources of evidence and relied mainly on clinical notes and what the patient said. If, however, you were planning for a child or a person who lacked capacity, you may have identified that you relied on what their family told you about their needs and preferences.

Conclusion

Ethical and moral theories and principles are useful for directing decision-making and actions, but they can also conflict with each other, producing moral and ethical dilemmas for the nurse. Clinical reasoning can help to problem-solve these dilemmas, but in itself will never be wholly satisfactory or entirely meet a person's needs. It is important for you to recognise this as a part of professional practice and an area for reflection in order to sustain further learning and develop your future practice.

Chapter summary

This chapter has explored some of the main ethical theories and principles that underpin nursing practice. These have been illustrated through case studies representing some common practice problems. You have been asked to explore critically and reflect on some of the issues raised. In so doing, you will have been able to identify some problems with translating ethical theory into ethical practice. Using this knowledge will enable you to better assess, plan, implement and evaluate patient care. Of course, understanding how to use these tools to make decisions is hard for any nurse, let alone a student. Approaches to clinical decision-making are addressed in some detail in Chapter 9, during which you should consider the lessons learnt in the previous chapters of this book.

Activities: brief outline answers

Activity 8.1 Critical thinking (page 135)

Ordinarily, we do not lie to people in the health and social care setting because it is important to treat people as autonomous equals, and because lying will undermine people's faith in health and social care professionals in the long term when the lie is uncovered. In this case, however, Pearl is unable to make sense of the world in which she lives, and her thinking that Ken is dead will only continue to upset her every time she is told. It would seem reasonable, therefore, to reassure her that he is coming later, if only to help her manage her distress and maximise her happiness.

Activity 8.2 Reflection (page 136)

It is likely that you would have considered the code of professional standards of practice and behaviour for nurses, midwives and nursing associates (NMC, 2018b), which states that you must: 'treat people with kindness, respect and compassion' and 'stay objective and have clear professional boundaries at all times with people in your care', as well as 'make sure you do not express your personal beliefs (including political, religious or moral beliefs) to people in an inappropriate way'. This means whatever your personal opinions and prejudices, you must not allow these to affect the way in which you treat an individual who is in your care. You may have identified situations where this might be personally difficult for you. In doing so, it is also important to consider strategies that will help you to overcome these difficulties and to meet and uphold the code within your practice at all times.

Activity 8.3 Critical thinking (page 139)

William's autonomy is affected by him not knowing where he is and therefore being unable to make informed decisions about whether he stays or goes. In addition, his wife is trying to make decisions for him. The Mental Capacity Act 2005 identifies that even if he is not able to make complex decisions, for example about his care arrangements when he goes home, he should nevertheless be consulted on simpler things (e.g. what he wishes to eat and drink, whether he wants to wash or get dressed, and what he wants to do with his day). It will be important for the healthcare team to determine whether William's decision-making capacity is temporarily or permanently affected. They will also need to consider who can make decisions on his behalf legally (i.e. who has lasting power of attorney or has been appointed by the court of protection as his deputy). A further consideration that you might have thought about is the relationship between William and his wife, Marjorie. Has she an agenda for wanting to take over and make decisions for him? Is this part of their normal relationship? The nurse is demonstrating courage in asking Marjorie to wait elsewhere with a cup of tea. The nurse is using communication to assess what William really perceives of the situation and is demonstrating care in this approach.

Activity 8.4 Critical thinking (page 144)

Your list of what Nancy needs to consider could have included:

- Sybil's autonomy in terms of (allegedly) being locked in her room;
- Sybil's mental capacity;
- the involvement of Sybil's grandson and his collusion;
- Sybil's confidentiality; and
- issues of beneficence and non-maleficence, in terms of trying to protect Sybil from being conned and losing all her money, as well as considering the relationship between Sybil and her daughter, Gloria, and grandson, Luke.

Nancy first needs to speak to Gloria to find out some background of what is going on at home. In doing so, she is not breaking Sybil's confidentiality. Nancy also needs to consider and assess Sybil's mental capacity and the organisational adult and child protection procedures. If she has concerns within these areas, she can then draw on these procedures, particularly as Sybil appears to be a vulnerable adult. Nancy could involve a social worker to help her with this.

Further reading

Beauchamp, T and Childress, J (2013) *Principles of Biomedical Ethics* (7th edn). Oxford: Oxford University Press.

This is perhaps the best-known ethical textbook in use on modern healthcare.

Ellis, P (2020) *Understanding Ethics for Nursing Students* (3rd edn). London: SAGE.

This book sets out how ethics can be approached deductively and inductively, and how students can use reflective techniques to enhance their ethical knowledge and understanding.

Rahman, S and Myers, R (2019) *Courage in Healthcare: A Necessary Virtue or a Warning Sign?* London: SAGE.

A book that challenges us to be courageous in supporting ethical healthcare delivery.

Seedhouse, D and Peutherer, V (2020) *Using Personal Judgement in Nursing and Healthcare.* London: SAGE.

This book explores ethical questions in healthcare from a practical standpoint.

Useful websites

www.nmc-uk.org

The website of the Nursing and Midwifery Council, where you can find a great deal of professional information, including the latest guidance on the code of conduct for nurses, midwives and nursing associates.

https://www.gov.uk/government/publications/wellbeing-in-mental-health-applying-all-our-health/wellbeing-in-mental-health-applying-all-our-health

This website provides guidance to health and social care professionals on mental capacity issues and mental health services.

https://www.scie.org.uk/atoz/getresultsbyletter?letter=M

The website for the Social Care Institute for Excellence has various pages dedicated to mental health, with information about government policies and best practice accessible from this page within their resources and services page.

http://jima.imana.org/article/viewFile/5245/38_3-3

This PDF download will help you to understand how different religions view ethics differently.

Chapter 9 · Patient assessment and decision-making

Mooi Standing

Platform 6: Improving safety and quality of care

At the point of registration, the registered nurse will be able to:

6.7   understand how the quality and effectiveness of nursing care can be evaluated in practice, and demonstrate how to use service delivery evaluation and audit findings to bring about continuous improvement.

Platform 7: Coordinating care

At the point of registration, the registered nurse will be able to:

7.9   facilitate equitable access to healthcare for people who are vulnerable or have a disability, demonstrate the ability to advocate on their behalf when required, and make necessary reasonable adjustments to the assessment, planning and delivery of their care.

Chapter aims

After reading this chapter, you will be able to:

- describe how patient assessment influences clinical decisions and interventions;
- appreciate the uncertainties, challenges and changing nature of health problems and preventative healthcare;
- identify strengths and weaknesses of intuitive versus analytical clinical judgement;
- apply cognitive continuum theory – nine modes of practice – to assessment and care;
- apply a matrix model – ten perceptions of decision-making – to assessment and care; and
- apply a 'PERSON' evaluation tool to assessment and decision-making in nursing care.

Introduction

Without accurate assessment of health problems, any decisions made about a person's care are likely to be unsafe and ineffective. Assessment, clinical judgement and decision-making are therefore closely linked because accurate identification of health problems needs to go hand in hand with delivering safe and effective nursing interventions. Chapters 1–8 showed how assessment involves gathering relevant information from various sources (e.g. what patients tell you, research evidence) in order to diagnose health problems, and then plan ethical, holistic nursing care (for individuals and communities) to address related health needs and prevent the problems recurring if possible. Using case studies, this chapter relates assessment of health problems to the clinical judgement, decision-making and interventions used to tackle them. Relevant theory and research, including cognitive continuum theory – nine modes of practice – and a matrix model – ten perceptions of clinical decision-making (Standing, 2010, 2023) – are applied to patient assessment. Finally, a 'PERSON' evaluation tool (Standing, 2023), developed in response to criticisms of nursing practice in the Francis Report (Francis, 2013), is applied to review and enhance patient assessment and decision-making in person-centred nursing care.

Assessment, clinical judgement, decision-making and healthcare interventions

The following case study highlights the interrelationship between assessment, clinical judgement, decision-making in nursing and interprofessional healthcare interventions.

Case study: Assessing Angela's ear complaint and deciding what to do about it

Angela, aged 48, is a police chief inspector. Part of her personal hygiene regime involves cleaning the inside of her ears with cotton buds. There are signs on the packaging warning against inserting them in ears, but Angela feels uncomfortable when she senses her ears need cleaning and this is the best method she has found to do so. One day, a cotton bud detaches itself and gets stuck inside her left ear. In trying to get it out, Angela pushes it further inside, increasing her discomfort. She takes paracetamol tablets every four hours to help control the pain.

Two days later, Angela cannot bear the constant irritation and pain anymore, so goes to see her GP. He uses an auroscope to examine her ear and sees the bud, but is unable to remove it. He refers Angela to the practice nurse (trained in electrical ear irrigation) for the removal of a 'foreign body' in her left ear. However, the device is in need of repair, so the nurse advises Angela to go to the local minor injury unit (MIU).

Kim is a first-year nursing student observing Nigel, a nurse practitioner at the MIU, who is sitting behind a desk in the consulting room while Angela explains what the problem is. Nigel gets up and examines her ear with an auroscope but cannot see anything that should not be there. Kim notices that Angela is getting irritated when she says, 'It has been there for the last two days. It is hurting my ear. It's making me feel dizzy and I cannot concentrate on my work. My GP saw it this morning and said it could be removed, so if you are unable to see it, surely you can still irrigate the ear and then it might come out?'

Kim senses that Nigel might feel his competence is being challenged. He asks Angela whether the GP used an auroscope like he did to examine her. An argument ensues as Angela champions the GP's expertise, Nigel claims that he is also a qualified medical practitioner, and Angela retorts that he is a nurse, not a doctor. Kim feels torn between respecting her senior colleague and sensing that Angela is not well.

Nigel asks Helen, a nurse practitioner colleague, to examine Angela's ear (using an auroscope), and she states that she can see no foreign object. Nigel tells Angela they can find nothing wrong so they will not be irrigating her ear. Angela leaves the MIU (after filling in an evaluation form where she is very critical of the care received) feeling very frustrated because she does not feel any better but has been told there is nothing wrong. She contacts the surgery and is offered an urgent appointment with a different GP. He cannot see any foreign body, but he notices that the ear is very inflamed, prescribes antibiotics (by mouth), and refers Angela to an ear, nose and throat (ENT) clinic. The ENT consultant confirms there is no foreign body in her left ear ('the cotton bud must have fallen out') but that her ear remains infected. He informs Angela that ear irrigation is not recommended for ear infections and prescribes antibiotic ear drops. He advises Angela not to use cotton buds any more, but to use wax-softening ear drops to clean her ears in future. One week later, Angela feels much better.

Angela's case study shows how a seemingly innocuous event such as a cotton bud getting stuck in a person's ear can result in pain, discomfort, irritability and infection (which, if not treated, could cause more serious problems such as deafness). The case study also conveys how many people can be involved in one person's care in a short space of time, and the variations in their assessment of the health problem and what they did about it. Activity 9.1 gives you a structure to guide your reflection about Angela's case study so that you can appreciate some of the challenges and uncertainties of patient assessment and related healthcare interventions.

Activity 9.1   Critical thinking and reflection

The purpose of this activity is to get you involved in exploring some of the issues discussed, identifying different ways that Angela's problem was assessed and treated, and for you to become more aware of the interrelationships between assessment, clinical judgement and decision-making. Read the case study again and then complete the table by summarising how each person diagnosed (defined) the problem and what action they decided was necessary to resolve the problem.

Person doing assessment	Problems they identified	Their decision-making/ action
Angela		
First GP		
Practice nurse		
Nigel (nurse practitioner)		

(Continued)

(Continued)

Person doing assessment	Problems they identified	Their decision-making/ action
Helen (nurse practitioner)		
Kim (student nurse)		
Second GP		
ENT consultant		

An outline answer is given at the end of the chapter.

Activity 9.1 illustrates the challenges and uncertainties in trying to reach an accurate diagnosis of a health problem and deciding the best course of action to take. In Angela's case study, the varied assessments and related clinical decision-making fall into three main groups, as shown in Table 9.1.

	Assessment and diagnosis	Clinical decision-making and action
1	Cotton bud/foreign body in left ear causing pain and discomfort	Remove foreign body from left ear
2	No foreign body in left ear and no health problem evident	No treatment required
3	Inflammation and infection in left ear causing pain and discomfort	Prescribe antibiotics to kill the bacteria causing the infection and thereby relieve symptoms

Table 9.1 Assessments and resulting decision-making

Each person assessing Angela's health problem used information (e.g. from what Angela reported, general observations and examination of her left ear) to make a decision based on the evidence available to them. The fact that they reached different diagnoses enables us to reach the following conclusions:

- Assessment, clinical judgement and decision-making is not an exact science.
- Healthcare practitioners have different sets of skills and may view problems differently.
- The potential for them to make errors means that nurses and doctors need to assess risks carefully regarding their proposed interventions. For example, Nigel missed signs of infection, but he was right not to irrigate the ear when he saw no reason to, because irrigation, although safer than ear syringing, can sometimes cause damage, especially if the ear is infected.
- Health problems are not static: they can clear up, stay the same, get worse or change. For example, the cotton bud causing discomfort apparently fell out but Angela still had an ear infection.
- Due to their changeable nature, health problems need to be continuously reassessed so that clinical judgement, decision-making and related interventions can be adjusted as needs be.

A flow chart rounds off this section, summarising the interrelationships between assessment of problems, diagnosis, clinical judgement, decision-making and healthcare interventions (see Figure 9.1). In Activity 9.2, you are asked to discuss and apply this flow chart to clinical practice.

Person presents with a health problem ←
↓
Healthcare practitioner uses clinical judgement to assess and diagnose problem
↓
Clinical judgement applies intuition, reflection and critical thinking skills
↓
Clinical judgement relates provisional diagnosis to various possible care options
↓
Care options identified through clinical judgement inform decision-making
↓
Clinical decision-making selects best option to deliver healthcare interventions
↓
Healthcare interventions are used to resolve problems or make them more bearable
↓
Person's health is hopefully improved/possibly unchanged/may deteriorate
↓
Evaluation prompts the end of/continuation of/reassessment of planned care
↓
The above process is repeated as necessary to resolve problems fully where possible

Figure 9.1   Assessment, clinical judgement, decision-making and healthcare interventions

Activity 9.2   Reflection and teamwork

The aim of this activity is to reinforce your understanding of the interrelationships between assessment, diagnosis, clinical judgement, decision-making and healthcare interventions. It also encourages you to appreciate teamwork in assessment and clinical decision-making.

Get together with some colleagues and work through the flow chart in Figure 9.1, thinking of examples from your combined experiences of practice placements. Remember how in Angela's case study, many different health professionals were involved, so try to incorporate the contributions of everyone concerned in the examples of patient assessment you and your colleagues identify. See if you can tease out different ways that they may have diagnosed a person's health problem and any differences in their clinical decision-making and interventions. Reflect on why this might have been so with reference to the various types of evidence on which they may have based their clinical judgement and decision-making. Review the effectiveness of interventions used in terms of patient outcomes, and how this influenced subsequent clinical decision-making. Finally, reflect on what you have learned from the activity and what aspects of the process described in the flow chart you feel you need to learn more about. See if you and your colleagues can help each other understand any issues a little better and/or agree plans to find out more.

As this activity is for you and your colleagues to discuss and learn from, no outline answer is given.

Applying decision theory and research to patient assessment and healthcare

Standing (2010) applied cognitive continuum theory to nursing and healthcare using nine modes of practice (mentioned in Chapter 2), used in Table 9.2 to review decisions in Angela's case study.

Nine modes	Examples of decision-making in Angela's case study of practice
Intuitive judgement	Angela felt it was OK to use cotton buds to clean her ear despite warnings against doing so; Kim sensed that Angela was not well when she became irritated.
Reflective judgement	Kim reflected on feeling torn between respecting senior colleague Nigel and empathising with Angela.
Patient and peer-aided judgement	Angela explained the problem to practitioners and described her symptoms (e.g. pain); they referred Angela to other practitioners (e.g. Nigel asked Helen to examine the ear).
System-aided judgement	Special equipment (auroscope) used to examine ears; systematic problem-solving approach adopted by all.
Critical review of experiential and research evidence	(a) Angela was critical of the care she received in the MIU. (b) The second GP and ENT consultant recognised signs of infection and knew which antibiotics to prescribe as treatment.
Action research and clinical audit	(a) Angela completed an evaluation form in the MIU to give feedback on aspects of care that she felt were poor; faulty electrical ear irrigation device needs repair at surgery. (b) ENT consultant advises Angela to stop putting cotton buds in her ears and to clean them with ear drops instead.
Qualitative research	(a) Angela's experience of care is a qualitative case study. (b) Kim's reflections on what she has learned from her experiences could be written up and published one day.
Survey research	Review of electrical ear irrigation indicates it is safer than ear syringing, but it still carries risks (e.g. damaging the eardrum if pressure is excessive or causing infection).
Experimental research	The antibiotics prescribed are developed and tested through scientific research and clinical trials.

Table 9.2 Nine modes of practice applied to Angela's case study

As you can see above, each of the nine modes of practice can be applied to review the decisions referred to in Angela's case study. This shows the wide range of knowledge and evidence that nurses and other practitioners draw upon in their clinical judgement and decision-making. Cognitive continuum theory of judgement and decision-making combines the two opposing extremes of *intuitive human judgement*, which is informed by a person's own subjective experience, versus *analytical decision-making*, which is informed by objective, scientific research (Hammond, 1996). The nine modes of practice show how judgement and decision-making can contain varying amounts of intuition and analysis, ranging from a 'gut feeling' about someone to giving medicine developed by scientific research and clinical trials.

Ideally, you don't have a favourite mode of practice that you stick to regardless of the circumstances. Intuition is invaluable when you have to make 'on-the-spot' decisions to react quickly when necessary, but if you rely too much on intuition you are likely to ignore important research evidence (e.g. Angela ignored the warning not to put a cotton bud in her ear). Analysis is invaluable when you have the time to research and plan evidence-based care, but if you rely too much on analysis you are likely to ignore important sensory or emotional information cues (e.g. Nigel focused on the absence of a cotton bud and did not notice the inflammation or acknowledge that Angela had a problem; he was also unaware of how his verbal and non-verbal communication style appeared to make things worse).

Clinical decision-making in nursing and healthcare can also make the difference between a person surviving or dying from an illness or injury, so it is vital that clinical judgement and decision-making is accurate in diagnosing problems and delivering safe and effective care. However, the case study showed that it is not an exact science, and human error can lead to important information (e.g. signs and symptoms of ill health) being missed or misinterpreted. This is why it makes sense to research clinical decision-making in order to learn more about it, develop better skills and competence, and reduce the likelihood of errors and mistakes occurring.

Each of the nine modes of practice has strengths and weaknesses, and the idea is to use the most appropriate one to match the nature of the problem you are about to tackle. To be able to do this, you need to develop knowledge and skills in all nine modes of practice. The next section will develop your understanding a bit more by asking you to apply the nine modes of practice to a case study regarding a nursing student's experience of patient assessment.

Applying the nine modes of practice to a nursing student's patient assessment

As a student nurse, you can rightly expect to receive guidance and role modelling in decision-making from registered nurses, practice supervisors and other health professionals. However, unless you go about in a permanent trance, you are making decisions independently every moment of your waking life, including during practice placements, as the following case study shows.

Case study: Assessing Vicky's complaint of being 'stressed out' and deciding what to do

Marion is a second-year nursing student doing a community placement. It includes working with a school nurse who looks after pupils' health needs (e.g. first aid, health education, support, advice, immunisation checks) at a large comprehensive school. Vicky, age 14, goes to the school nurse's office and asks Marion if she can give her something for her 'nerves'. Marion explains that she is not the nurse, who should be back in 20 minutes, and asks Vicky if she wants to wait or come back. Vicky opts to stay and tells Marion that she hates coming to school and that it's 'stressing her out'. Marion asks if there is anything in particular that she finds stressful about school. Vicky describes feeling frightened and embarrassed because Sue, an older pupil, 'has a crush' on her, keeps trying to kiss her on the lips, follows her around both at school and on the way home, and will not stop stalking her despite Vicky saying, 'Stay away from me'. When Vicky rejected her advances, Sue apparently got angry and told her parents that a head wound she received (during a fight with a young woman who kicked her when she was lying on the floor) was caused by Vicky attacking her. Sue's parents then accosted Vicky and her mum in their car outside an ice-skating club (where they knew Vicky went), verbally abused them, kicked the car, broke a door mirror, and punched Vicky's mum when she told them to stop. Vicky says she cannot sleep, is 'off her food', feels sick all the time, is really scared of Sue, and wants Marion to give her something that will 'make it all go away'.

While Vicky is describing these very disturbing events, Marion wonders what she has let herself in for as she feels completely out of her depth. Just then, she remembers a lecture on safeguarding vulnerable people and she realises that she is duty-bound to tell the school nurse what Vicky has said. The school nurse returns to the office and Marion briefs her about how she has handled Vicky's request for help, and the gist of her problems. The school nurse says Marion has done well to enable Vicky to talk, and it is important to keep a record of this and report the matter to the head teacher, Vicky's teacher, parents and GP after she has spoken to Vicky.

Vicky's case study shows that you never quite know what might happen during your clinical placements. When something unexpected does happen, you often have to think on your feet and make a decision on the spot without the benefit of advice from a senior colleague or the opportunity to research how you should respond. Activity 9.3 asks you to review Marion's decision-making in caring for Vicky with reference to Standing's nine modes of practice.

Activity 9.3   Critical thinking and decision-making

The purpose of this activity is to give you some practice in applying decision theory to patient assessment and decision-making. Look back at how the nine modes of practice were used to review decision-making in Angela's case study, and then try to apply as many of the nine modes you think are appropriate to the decision-making evident in Vicky's case study.

Nine modes of practice	Examples of decision-making in Vicky's case study
Intuitive judgement	
Reflective judgement	
Patient and peer-aided judgement	
System-aided judgement	
Critical review of experiential and research evidence	
Action research and clinical audit	
Qualitative research	
Survey research	
Experimental research	

An outline answer is given at the end of the chapter.

A matrix model of nursing students' perceptions of clinical decision-making

Both Angela's and Vicky's case studies provide a glimpse of what it is like to be a student nurse (Kim and Marion) during practice placements, observing, reflecting on experience, and developing skills in patient assessment, clinical judgement and decision-making. A research study of nursing students' reflections on developing decision-making skills created a matrix model describing ten perceptions (key aspects) of clinical decision-making in nursing (Standing, 2023). Table 9.3 lists the ten perceptions of decision-making identified by the nursing students in Standing's research study, together with a brief description of each one.

Collaborative	Consulting with patients, relatives, nurses, practice supervisors and health professionals to inform relevant patient-centred decisions.
Observation	Use of senses to assess patients' physical and mental health, monitor vital signs, review investigations, record responses to nursing/healthcare interventions and report any concerns.

(Continued)

Table 9.3   (Continued)

Systematic	Using critical thinking and problem-solving skills to assess problems, set goals, deliver care and evaluate outcomes.
Standardised	Application of NHS trust policies, procedures and care plans, research evidence-based clinical guidelines and assessment tools.
Prioritising	Risk assessment and management to avoid causing harm to any patient, targeting care on those with more serious problems first, and safeguarding the vulnerable (e.g. physical or mental disability).
Experience and intuition	Recognising similarities and differences in current and previous situations, being guided by what worked before, not repeating mistakes, or realising you may lack the experience to make a decision.
Reflective	Reviewing events as they happen (reflection in action) or looking back (reflection on action) for insight into the best course of action.
Ethical sensitivity	Applying ethical principles (autonomy, justice, beneficence, non-maleficence) to ensure patients' human rights are respected (e.g. maintaining confidentiality, gaining informed consent to procedures).
Accountability	Being answerable to patients, public, NHS trusts, Nursing and Midwifery Council and the legal system for the consequences of your actions and being able to explain, justify and defend your decisions when asked to do so.
Confidence	Self-assurance from experience and achievements and professional assurance that give patients and colleagues confidence in you.

Table 9.3   Matrix model: ten perceptions of clinical decision-making in nursing

Activity 9.4   Reflection

Take a moment to think about the matrix model – the ten perceptions of clinical decision-making in nursing. This description of clinical decision-making came from pooling nursing students' reflections of their experiences in clinical practice over a four-year period, which included their first year as registered nurses. Does it tally with your experience? Can you relate to the different aspects of decision-making that are identified? Can you think of any other aspects that are not incorporated in the matrix model? How do you think it compares to the cognitive continuum theory – the nine modes of practice?

As this is for your own reflection, no outline answer is provided.

Comparing the nine modes of practice and ten perceptions of clinical decision-making

The ten perceptions of decision-making, like the nine modes of practice, is an evidence-based tool to guide and evaluate patient assessment, clinical judgement and decision-making. Both describe a range of knowledge and skills, and there are some clear similarities between them, as shown below.

Similarities in some of the modes of practice and perceptions of clinical decision-making

Modes of practice	Perceptions of clinical decision-making
Intuitive judgement	Experience and intuition
Reflective judgement	Reflective
Patient and peer-aided judgement	Collaborative
System-aided judgement	Systematic
Action research and clinical audit	Standardised

Due to their similarity, applying the above modes of practice and perceptions of decision-making to guide or review patient assessment would more or less cover the same ground. For example, if – when doing Activity 9.3 – you interpreted Marion's rapport with Vicky as an example of 'patient and peer-aided judgement', it would also be an example of 'collaborative' clinical decision-making if you were applying the matrix model. However, the other four modes of practice are more clearly research-focused (critical review of experiential and research evidence, qualitative, survey and experimental research). In contrast, the other five perceptions of decision-making are more clearly clinically focused (observation, prioritising, ethical sensitivity, accountability and confidence). To get an idea of what these perceptions of decision-making have to offer, it is worth seeing what light they cast on Vicky's case study (see Table 9.4).

Perceptions of clinical decision-making	Examples of decision-making in Vicky's case study
Observation	Marion observed that Vicky wanted something to make the stress go away, that she was prepared to wait to see the school nurse, that she was responsive to Marion asking probing questions about what might have led to her feeling stressed at school, and that – given her account of events – it was understandable that she should feel stressed out.
Prioritising	Marion and the school nurse identified that taking steps to protect Vicky from abuse and to ensure her safety was the main priority.
Ethical sensitivity	Marion respected Vicky's autonomy in choosing to tell someone about her problem; she was aware of the sensitive and confidential nature of their discussion while realising she had a duty to report it to the appropriate authorities; her actions appeared to help Vicky (beneficence) explain what was upsetting her, and help protect her from the alleged bullying, harassment and intimidation (maleficence) by Sue in the foreseeable future.

(Continued)

Table 9.4   (Continued)

Perceptions of clinical decision-making	Examples of decision-making in Vicky's case study
Accountability	Marion and the school nurse realised that the school has a duty to provide a safe environment for pupils and to take action where risks are identified; they also had to document what had happened as they might be called upon to explain and justify their actions.
Confidence	Marion's confidence was initially shaken when she found out the seriousness of Vicky's problems; she recovered her composure by focusing on safeguarding Vicky against further potential abuse, and her confidence was boosted when the school nurse said she did well.

Table 9.4   Perceptions of clinical decision-making applied to Vicky's case study

Activity 9.5   Critical thinking and decision-making

Take a moment to look back at Activity 9.3, where you applied the nine modes of practice to review patient assessment in Vicky's case study. Now look at the above application of five perceptions of decision-making and reflect on whether they help to identify any aspects of patient assessment that you did not find out using the nine modes of practice.

As this is for your own reflection, no outline answer is provided.

Both cognitive continuum theory and the matrix model offer evidence-based frameworks to guide, review and develop clinical judgement and decision-making in patient assessment. The matrix model is particularly relevant in pre-registration nurse education as the ten perceptions of decision-making come from nursing students' reflections on their clinical experiences. It also complements previous chapters by encouraging a cooperative, person-centred, holistic (bio-psycho-social-spiritual), ethical and health-promoting approach to patient assessment.

Applying the matrix model to patient assessment, clinical decision-making and healthcare

Successfully carrying out person-centred, holistic patient assessment to inform clinical decision-making in delivering safe and effective healthcare sounds lovely in theory, but making it happen in reality is very challenging. As health professionals become more technically skilled, their clinical focus tends to narrow on specific aspects of care, and this can go against seeing patients as unique individuals. The next case study shows the problems that can occur when this happens.

Case study: A lesson in patient assessment and holistic care from Francis and his family

Francis, age 39, has received mental health care for 20 years since he was diagnosed as suffering from paranoid schizophrenia during his first year at university. When Francis is well, he is a shy, artistic, thoughtful and placid person. When unwell, he is convinced that people want to harm him (when they don't), and these false beliefs (delusions of persecution) are resistant to reason or evidence that challenges them. He may also hear voices (auditory hallucinations), which can make him agitated and aggressive. Francis's mental health has been stabilised through medication (e.g. clozapine, an antipsychotic drug) and support from his family and community agencies. His mum, Elizabeth, and dad, Jeffrey, live in the same town and encourage Francis to visit or stay with them whenever he wishes. The parents never go away on holiday together to make sure that one of them is always available if he needs them. He has a younger brother, James, living 60 miles away, who he likes to talk to on the phone.

Two months ago, Francis found that he could not move his left arm or feel his fingers, so he went to the GP surgery. He saw a GP, who did not detect that anything was wrong. A few days later, Jeffrey saw Francis and was worried about his inability to move his left arm. Jeffrey took Francis to an out-of-hours service at a local NHS trust hospital, where the duty GP said Francis might benefit from physiotherapy, but no referral was made. A week later, there was no change. Elizabeth was so concerned that she took Francis to see the GP and insisted that something was done to find out why he could not move his left arm. The GP referred Francis to have a computed tomography (CT) scan to check for problems.

On the day of the scan, Elizabeth asked Francis to take a lorazepam tablet (as prescribed) to reduce his anxiety, she accompanied him to the hospital and the CT scan was carried out. They were not told the result, but a week later Francis got a letter with an urgent appointment for a magnetic resonance imaging (MRI) scan. No reason was given, and this made Francis very anxious.

Elizabeth went to see the GP to ask for an explanation and was told the CT scan showed an abnormality in Francis's brain that needed further investigation. She prepared and accompanied Francis for the MRI scan (as she had done for the CT scan) and it was carried out without incident. They were not told the result, but a week later Francis got a telephone call from the GP asking him to pick up a referral letter from the surgery and take it to the emergency care unit of the local hospital for him to be admitted.

Francis was upset and anxious and he called his mother. Elizabeth was surprised the GP did not let her know about this so that she might support Francis. She took him to the emergency care unit, where a consultant informed them that the MRI scan indicated Francis had had a stroke (also called a cerebrovascular accident, CVA) due to haemorrhaging (bleeding) in his brain. Francis was transferred to a ward that assessed and treated patients with strokes.

(Continued)

(Continued)

Francis was admitted to the stroke ward by Julie, a third-year nursing student. The ward used an integrated care pathway to guide and coordinate the multidisciplinary healthcare team in key aspects of assessment and treatment of patients who had suffered from a stroke. Julie's initial assessment of Francis focused on identifying any impairment of sensation and movement in Francis's limbs, particularly in his left arm, and how long this had been so. She did not ask about Francis's previous medical history. Julie informed Francis that he would need to have another MRI scan, 'probably sometime tomorrow'.

The next day, Francis was getting increasingly anxious and distressed. He knew Elizabeth was at work, so he phoned James and began crying, saying, 'I don't know what is going on'. James assured Francis that he would drive down to see him in the afternoon. In the meantime, a hospital porter asked Francis to sit in a wheelchair and took him to have his second MRI scan. The nurses were busy at the time and no one explained to Francis where he was being taken. At the MRI unit, Francis was highly anxious, very distressed and agitated. He started swearing and screaming at the staff not to touch him when they tried to do the MRI scan.

Francis was taken back to the ward. When James arrived, he was still agitated and bad-tempered, shouting and swearing at the nurses, who were unsure how to deal with him. He complained of pain in his left arm, which was bruised from unsuccessful attempts to insert an intravenous line in the MRI unit. James tried to calm Francis down, but he was too upset, and so James called their mother. Elizabeth came straight away, and she managed to comfort Francis and get him to relax a little bit, assuring him that nobody there really wanted to hurt him. The next day, Elizabeth got the consultant to agree to discharge Francis to the care of his family, who would prepare and accompany him for further tests or treatments as an outpatient.

Francis's case study provides a graphic account of how important accurate patient assessment is and how difficult it can sometimes be for doctors and nurses to achieve this. When things do not go as well as they should, it is vital to learn from the experience in order to improve. Francis and his family demonstrated many of the skills in person-centred, holistic patient assessment and care that nurses and other health professionals can learn from, as shown in Table 9.5.

Collaborative	(a) Francis informed the GP about his arm problem. (b) Jeffrey took Francis for a second opinion from a GP at the out-of-hours service. (c) James came to support Francis when he was distressed.
Observation	Francis and his parents saw that he had lost the ability to move his left arm, recognised that it needed investigation and alerted the GP.
Systematic	Elizabeth carefully prepared Francis for the CT and MRI scans by explaining what they were for, accompanying him to the hospital and supporting him during procedures to help relieve his anxiety.

Standardised	(a) Francis continued taking prescribed antipsychotic medication. (b) Elizabeth also asked him to take prescribed lorazepam tablets on the day of the scan to help control and relieve his anxiety.
Prioritising	When Francis's weakness in his left arm did not improve, Elizabeth insisted that the GP arrange for the problem to be investigated.
Experience and intuition	Francis and his family sensed that something was physically wrong with him despite not knowing that he had had a stroke at that time.
Reflective	Francis's family were aware of his mental fragility if stressed, and realised that they had to support and nurse him through the investigations and procedures to avoid him becoming disturbed.
Ethical sensitivity	(a) Francis's family respected his autonomy – when he said something was wrong with his arm, they believed him (and were right to). (b) They applied beneficence by being very caring towards him.
Accountability	(a) Francis's family took responsibility for arranging for his discharge from hospital because the poor care he received was upsetting him. (b) They looked after him at home while supporting him during further investigations and treatment for the stroke as an outpatient.
Confidence	(a) Francis had confidence in his family's ability to help him because they saw beyond his diagnosis of paranoid schizophrenia and knew him as a unique person whom they loved and cared for. (b) His family knew that while he was taking antipsychotic medication, Francis was receptive to their attempts to explain things and help him.

Table 9.5   Ten perceptions of clinical decision-making applied by Francis and his family

Francis's case study reveals the challenges in applying the theory of person-centred, holistic assessment and care to practice. Francis's medical history of long-term mental illness appears to have got in the way of doctors and nurses being attentive to his physical and psychological needs. This is evident in the initial failure to take his physical complaint about not being able to move his arm seriously. Once it was clear that Francis had suffered a stroke, he was not given the care and psychological support in hospital that anyone would be entitled to receive. Francis and his family demonstrated how he should have been cared for by the doctors and nurses. This emphasises the importance of being open-minded, carefully observing patients, communicating with them and taking note of what they say to ensure that assessment and related care decisions are relevant to their specific individual needs and preferences. Applying the matrix model to patient assessment, decision-making and care interventions in this way can help nurses to succeed in relating theory in person-centred, holistic care to the reality of clinical practice.

Applying a 'PERSON' evaluation tool in nursing

So far in this chapter, we have looked at the interrelationship between patient assessment, clinical judgement and decision-making and related nursing interventions. We also applied relevant theory and research findings to help identify, develop, understand and apply a range of key knowledge, skills and attitudes to patient assessment. As the above case study shows, healthcare professionals can make mistakes and patients suffer as a result. We therefore need to continually evaluate patient assessment, care plans and decision-making to identify where we can improve. Evaluating nursing decisions in assessing, planning and delivering patient care has been defined as follows:

A critical review of nursing decisions and associated care in: (i) addressing patients' rights, needs, problems and preferences; (ii) avoiding causing harm to patients; (iii) carrying out interventions that have beneficial outcomes for patients; (iv) applying relevant evidence, research and clinical guidelines to patient care; (v) identifying strengths and weaknesses of care provided; and (vi) considering the implications of the findings for continuing patient care and our own professional development and education needs as nurses.

(Standing, 2023)

This definition of what evaluating nursing decisions means was developed in response to the publication of the Francis Report in 2013. In this government commissioned Public Inquiry into NHS failings, led by Robert Francis QC (now Sir Robert Francis KC), unacceptable standards of care in an NHS trust whose priority was meeting certain health targets (e.g. quantity of patients processed) rather than the quality of care patients received, were reported. Patients' and relatives' concerns and complaints were ignored; unsafe, ineffective care with poor patient outcomes was allowed to continue for years; and healthcare professionals were discouraged from 'whistle-blowing' about this. Evaluating nursing decisions must therefore focus on patients' experiences and feedback about care they receive, and identify better ways of delivering safe and effective care that addresses their needs and health problems, prompting nurses to be open and honest in reviewing their actions and being committed to developing their clinical competence. A 'PERSON' evaluation tool was developed to address all of the points in the above definition, and this can be applied within all fields of nursing (adult, children's, mental health, learning disability). It also summarises professional standards of conduct that nurses must adhere to (NMC, 2018b). The 'PERSON' acronym stands for the following:

P = patient-centred

E = evidence-based

R = risks assessed and managed

S = safe and effective delivery of care

O = outcomes of care benefit the patient

N = nursing and midwifery strengths and weaknesses

In order to evaluate nursing decisions using each element of the 'PERSON' evaluation tool, a series of questions was devised for nurses to answer in reviewing the quality of care they have provided, as described in Table 9.6.

'PERSON' acronym	Answer questions to evaluate decisions
Patient-centred	Were different care options explained to the patient?
	Did the patient give consent before the intervention?
	How did the patient's opinion contribute to care plans?
	If for any reason the patient was unable to contribute to decisions, how were their rights safeguarded?
Evidence-based	What patient observations indicated a need for action?
	What corroborating evidence supports your assessment?
	What was the rationale for the selected intervention?
	What research evidence underpins the intervention?
Risks assessed and managed	What threats to the patient's health/well-being were there?
	What was done to ensure a safe healthcare environment?
	What procedure did you follow to control known risks?
	How did you escalate concerns if problems worsened?
Safe and effective delivery of care	What knowledge/skills/attitudes were applied to care?
	What prior experience did you have of this intervention?
	How was your competence to give care quality assured?
	How did you share information on the care you gave?
Outcomes of care benefit the patient	What was the patient's/relatives' feedback about care?
	To what extent were desired outcomes of care achieved?
	How do you think the patient benefited from this care?
	How will you address any negative outcomes of care?
Nursing and midwifery strengths and weaknesses	What did you learn from this experience of patient care?
	How did you justify public trust in your ability to care?
	On reflection, what could you have done differently?
	What are you doing to improve decision-making skills?

Table 9.6   Clinical decision-making 'PERSON' evaluation tool

Source: Standing (2023)

The 'PERSON' evaluation tool also incorporates relevant decision theory (nine modes of practice) and research (ten perceptions of clinical decision-making), discussed earlier in the chapter. For example, there is a strong emphasis on nurses respecting patients' human rights, collaborating with patients, colleagues and others, using observation and prioritising skills, and being systematic, reflective and accountable in delivering and critically reviewing patient care. Table 9.7 applies the 'PERSON' evaluation tool to review Marion's assessment of Vicky in the second case study.

Patient-centred
Were different care options explained to the patient? Marion gave Vicky the option of waiting or coming back in 20 minutes when the registered school nurse would be there.
Did the patient give consent before the intervention? Vicky chose to wait and voluntarily began telling Marion about her problems.
How did the patient's opinion contribute to care plans? Vicky wanted something to be done to help her deal with feeling 'stressed out'.
If for any reason the patient was unable to contribute to decisions, how were their rights safeguarded? Vicky is a vulnerable minor who reported being abused. To safeguard her, subsequent decisions would need to involve her parents, teachers and GP.
Evidence-based
What patient observations indicated a need for action? Vicky went to the school nurse's office seeking help, was not put off when she wasn't there, and she described physical and psychological symptoms associated with anxiety and stress in relation to her account of being intimidated and assaulted by Sue.
What corroborating evidence supports your assessment? Marion only had Vicky's account of events to go on at the time, but it did explain why she felt 'stressed out' and why she wanted help to deal with it.
What was the rationale for the selected intervention? Marion applied listening, communication and interpersonal skills in responding to Vicky's wish to talk about her problems and enabling her to do so.
What research evidence underpins the intervention? The communication and interpersonal skills that Marion applied echo the findings of research questions about what nursing students associated with being a nurse. Their conceptions of nursing included 'listening and being there', 'communicating' and being 'empathising and non-judgemental' (Standing, 2023).
Risks assessed and managed
What threats to the patient's health/well-being were there? Vicky's physical health was a concern as she indicated she was not eating properly/felt sick and said she had been verbally and physically assaulted. Her mental health was also a concern as she was frightened, anxious and felt unable to cope.
What was done to ensure a safe healthcare environment? The school nurse's office provided a place of safety for pupils to discuss personal and confidential issues affecting their health and well-being.
What procedure did you follow to control known risks? Marion made it clear to Vicky that she was not the school nurse, but that she would be back in 20 minutes. In this way, she acknowledged her limitations in competence (NMC, 2018b) and that the school nurse was supervising her clinical placement.
How did you escalate concerns if problems worsened? When it became clear that Vicky's problems were of a serious nature affecting her health and well-being both in and outside school, Marion realised that she was unable to resolve these issues herself and she had a duty to report this to the school nurse.

Safe and effective delivery of care

What knowledge/skills/attitudes were applied to care? In addition to the communication skills discussed above, Marion remembered a lecture regarding safeguarding, and this helped her to understand that Vicky is a vulnerable minor who needs to be protected from harm.

What prior experience did you have of this intervention? Marion had no experience of dealing with this challenging situation.

How was your competence to give care quality assured? Marion recognised that she was out of her depth given the seriousness of Vicky's problems, and that the school nurse needed to deal with it.

How did you share information on the care you gave? Marion informed the school nurse about how she had responded to Vicky's request for help and all the details of the problems that she described. The school nurse also asked Marion to write notes on what Vicky had told her as a formal record.

Outcomes of care benefit the patient

What was the patient's/relatives' feedback about care? The case study does not give details of Vicky's response to Marion's care. Her willingness to talk to Marion suggests that she felt comfortable doing so.

To what extent were desired outcomes of care achieved? Vicky wanted Marion to give her something to make the stress go away, suggesting that she was looking for medication to relieve anxiety, which Marion was not in a position to give. However, Marion's interventions helped to uncover the causes of Vicky's fear and anxiety, which laid the foundation for the alleged bullying and intimidation to be dealt with.

How do you think the patient benefitted from this care? It took a lot of courage for Vicky to confide in someone about her problems, and if Marion had not been welcoming and approachable Vicky might have gone away, not come back, had her sense of being victimised reinforced, and her problems unresolved.

How will you address any negative outcomes of care? While Marion coped well with the situation, being left on her own to deal with pupils' health problems poses risks that need to be managed more effectively in future (e.g. not being left alone or calling the school nurse to supervise or deal with problems).

Nursing and midwifery strengths and weaknesses

What did you learn from this experience of patient care? Marion gained valuable experience in communicating with Vicky to assess why she was feeling 'stressed out'. She was also able to apply the theory of safeguarding to clinical practice, which reinforced her understanding. The school nurse said that she had done well, and this helped to validate Marion's positive learning experience.

How did you justify public trust in your ability to care? Marion put her feelings of being shocked by what Vicky told her to one side in order to behave in a professional manner. She focused on what Vicky needed from her and recognised that she needed to tell the school nurse about this situation.

On reflection, what could you have done differently? The school nurse told Marion she needed to produce a written report of her interactions with Vicky. With hindsight, it would be helpful for Marion to get in the habit of making notes or filling in forms during assessments. This would help to structure interviews, ensure vital details are included, reduce recall errors, and aid accurate documentation.

What are you doing to improve decision-making skills? Marion is a second-year student, so she will continue to learn about decision-making skills during her nursing degree. She will also reflect on this episode of care and may incorporate this in her personal and professional development portfolio.

Table 9.7 Applying the 'PERSON' evaluation tool to review Marion's assessment of Vicky

Preventative healthcare assessment and decision-making

Each of the case studies in this chapter has involved nurses in caring for patients with physical and/or mental health problems affecting their activities of living and sense of well-being. Hence, focusing on treating people's ill health might seem unrelated to preventative healthcare since the current illness was not prevented. Nevertheless, as nurses we are required to apply principles of prevention in our assessment of patients, decision-making and nursing actions (see NMC proficiencies at the beginning of this chapter). However, our involvement with patients often results from a failure of primary prevention (preventing illness occurring), for example, in the first case study ignoring instructions not to insert cotton buds into ears to clean them, resulting in ear infection. Nurses do have opportunities for the early detection of health risks and timely intervention before they escalate into more serious health problems (secondary prevention). For example, in the second case study the school nurse took action to safeguard an anxious and frightened pupil who reported being abused by another pupil and her family. In caring for people with longer-term health issues, all carers have a duty to minimise further complications, help patients to manage their conditions, and support them in living satisfying lives as independently as possible (tertiary prevention). For example, in the third case study, the family of a vulnerable mental health patient who had suffered a cerebral vascular accident demonstrated how to communicate with him to reduce his anxiety and aggression that arose from his paralysis and fear of being harmed by healthcare staff.

Hence, promoting health and preventing illness are part and parcel of nurses' duty to assess patients' health needs and deciding what advice to give or action to take. Some nurses' roles and responsibilities are predominantly focused on preventative aspects of healthcare in the community, as the following case study illustrates.

Case study: Len's abdominal aortic aneurysm screening

Len, aged 65, was invited to his local health centre for abdominal aortic aneurysm (AAA) screening. The ultrasound scan showed Len has an AAA measuring 3cm. Holly, a vascular nurse practitioner, informs Len he has a small asymptomatic aneurysm, advises his GP to prescribe Len daily aspirin 75mg to slow growth of AAA, and advises Len to have 12-monthly AAA scans to check if it is getting bigger. For the first three years Len's AAA remains at 3cm, but in the next two years it increases to 3.7cm. Len and his wife Ruby are worried it is going to burst and Len will die prematurely. Holly sees Len and Ruby and explains that it is normal for AAAs to increase by a couple of mm per year and that 3 to 4.4cm is still classified as a small AAA. 4.5 to 5.4cm is a medium AAA, prompting more frequent, three-monthly scans. 5.5cm and above is classified as a large higher risk AAA, for which surgical intervention may be offered to prevent a rupture. Holly takes Len's blood pressure, which is normal, establishes that Len has not smoked for 45 years, and that he is now prescribed statins to manage his cholesterol level. Holly informs Len and Ruby that all this means that his AAA remains a relatively low risk and that continuing with 12-monthly AAA scanning will ensure appropriate further action can be taken if needed. Len and Ruby feel reassured his AAA will not just suddenly rupture as they had feared.

We can apply the PERSON evaluation tool to Len's case study, as follows:

[P] Patient-centred: The AAA screening service is voluntary so Len was free to choose to attend or not. It was made accessible for Len by arranging with his local health centre for the AAA scanning team to use their facilities on the day. When Len and Ruby were worried about the increased size of his AAA, Holly arranged to see them both, listen, and respond to their concerns with reassuring information.

[E] Evidence-based: Males aged 65 and over are more at risk of developing an AAA, which is why the NHS offers AAA screening to them (PHE, 2017). Len was found to have a small asymptomatic AAA. Ongoing monitoring and management of Len's AAA by Holly is informed by research-based clinical guidelines (NICE, 2020).

[R] Risks assessed and managed: A ruptured AAA is a medical emergency which only 20% of patients survive (NHS, 2021). Before losing consciousness, patients may report symptoms of acute abdominal or back pain. Larger AAAs are at greater risk of rupturing. If Len had not been screened, his small AAA would remain undetected. Regular monitoring of Len's AAA ensures preventative action can be taken if his AAA becomes so enlarged it is considered at risk of rupturing. Smoking weakens arterial walls, which increases AAA risks. Holly established that Len used to be a smoker but has not smoked for 45 years, thereby reducing this risk. High blood pressure increases AAA risks, which is why Holly checked Len's blood pressure and found it was normal. The build-up of atheroma (fatty cholesterol deposits) in the lining of arterial walls also weakens them, increasing AAA risks, which is why Holly checked this with Len, who confirmed that he was now prescribed statins to reduce his cholesterol level.

[S] Safe and effective delivery of care: Ultrasound scanning in AAA screening is a quick, non-invasive, reliable procedure carried out by trained technicians. They gave Len an AAA Surveillance card on which they recorded the measurement at each scan. Len was advised to carry it on him in case he needed medical attention. Holly wrote to Len's GP to inform them about the results of each scan which she copied to Len. She also gave Len her phone number to contact her with any concerns, which he and Ruby made use of.

[O] Outcomes of care benefit for the patient: Being informed of his AAA caused Len anxiety but he understood it meant he could be monitored, enabling action to be taken to prevent rupturing. Len and Ruby appreciated Holly making time to see them and respond to their concerns about the increased size of his AAA.

[N] Nursing & midwifery strengths and weaknesses: Holly reflected on how Len appeared fitter than most men attending AAA screening, highlighting the covert nature of some disease processes in people who seem healthy at first glance. Len's normal blood pressure and the apparent absence of lifestyle risk factors of smoking and obesity led Holly to conclude that Len's AAA might be due to genetic factors. As Len has a son, Holly advised Len and his GP that once his son turned 50 years of age, she recommended he be AAA screened due to the possible familial trait. This example of Holly's proactive preventative healthcare is a key nursing strength.

The above worked examples illustrate how the 'PERSON' evaluation tool offers a comprehensive framework to evaluate patient assessments, nursing decisions and associated preventative healthcare. It does so by incorporating relevant decision theory and research and standards within nurses' professional code of conduct. It takes on board recommendations of the Francis Report in quality-assuring safe and effective person-centred care, where nurses are open and honest in acknowledging errors and their development needs. It also addresses health policy priorities: (i) applying the 6Cs – care, compassion, competence, communication, courage and commitment as nurses (DH and NHS CB, 2012); and (ii) applying the NHS Long Term Care Plan as nurses in promoting health and preventing illness (NHS, 2019). It is recommended that you use this tool to guide and evaluate your decision-making and to structure your personal and professional development portfolios.

Chapter summary

This chapter has shown you how assessing health problems involves clinical judgement (intuition, reflection, critical thinking) in reaching a diagnosis and considering possible courses of action. Clinical decision-making is where a choice is made about which care intervention to use. Two frameworks, cognitive continuum theory (nine modes of practice) and a matrix model (ten perceptions of clinical decision-making), were offered to guide the development, application and review of clinical judgement and decision-making skills. A 'PERSON' evaluation tool to guide and evaluate assessment, care plans and nursing interventions was then discussed. The 'PERSON' evaluation tool is recommended for you to use as it incorporates relevant decision theory and research, the NMC code of conduct and current health policy priorities, and addresses the Francis Report recommendations. It also complements person-centred, holistic patient assessment, care planning and nursing interventions in preventative healthcare, which are advocated throughout this book.

Activities: brief outline answers

Activity 9.1   Critical thinking and reflection (page 153)

You may have included some of the following points:

Person doing assessment	Problems they identified	Their decision-making/action
Angela	Cotton bud stuck in left ear, pain, discomfort, dizziness, cannot concentrate on work, unable to bear it anymore	Try unsuccessfully to remove cotton bud, take paracetamol tablets to relieve pain, ask GP and nurses to remove it
First GP	Foreign body in left ear, pain and discomfort reported by Angela	Try unsuccessfully to remove it, refer to practice nurse for ear irrigation to remove it
Practice nurse	Foreign body in left ear, as advised by GP	Unable to do ear irrigation (equipment not working), refer Angela to the MIU
Nigel (nurse practitioner)	No foreign body in left ear, no health problem evident	(a) Request second opinion from nurse practitioner colleague; (b) refuse to do ear irrigation; (c) discharge Angela from MIU
Helen (nurse practitioner)	No foreign body in left ear	Attend to another patient
Kim (student nurse)	Angela was getting irritated, sensed that she was not well	Keep quiet and just observe, reflecting on feeling torn between respect for Nigel and empathising with Angela
Second GP	(a) No foreign body in left ear; (b) left ear inflamed and infected	Prescribe antibiotics (by mouth), refer to ENT
ENT consultant	(a) No foreign body in left ear; (b) left ear still appears infected	(a) Prescribe antibiotic ear drops; (b) confirm ear irrigation not appropriate; (c) give health promotion advice to Angela (i.e. stop putting cotton buds in ears, use ear drops instead)

Activity 9.3 Critical thinking and decision-making (page 159)

You may have included some of the following points:

Nine modes of practice	Examples of decision-making in Vicky's case study
Intuitive judgement	(a) Vicky felt unable to cope so she sought help. (b) Marion sensed that Vicky needed to talk to someone. (c) Marion felt 'completely out of her depth' at one point.
Reflective judgement	Just when Marion was thinking she did not know what she was doing, she remembered a safeguarding lecture, and realised she had a duty to report Vicky's problems to an appropriate authority (given that Vicky is a vulnerable minor, aged 14, who has reported being abused).
Patient and peer-aided judgement	(a) Marion did not send Vicky away (after she had gained the courage to speak to someone about her problem) and she enabled Vicky to tell her what was 'stressing her out'. (b) Marion reported the matter to the school nurse, which influenced her subsequent action (e.g. inform head teacher, explore issues further with Vicky).

(Continued)

(Continued)

Nine modes of practice	Examples of decision-making in Vicky's case study
System-aided judgement	(a) The school nursing service is part of the organisational structure of the school and pupils know they can seek help there for health-related problems. (b) Marion and the school nurse appeared to understand that they had a moral and legal duty to report Vicky's suspected abuse.
Critical review of experiential and research evidence	The school nurse gave Marion positive feedback for her role in enabling Vicky to talk about her problems.
Action research and clinical audit	(a) The school nurse was aware that formal records needed to be kept of what Vicky had said, which may be subject to official scrutiny. (b) The school nurse recognised that Vicky's suspected abuse requires further action to be taken by the head teacher, as well as Vicky's teacher, parents and GP, to ensure Vicky's safety at (and to and from) school.
Qualitative research	Vicky's experience of care by the school nursing service is a qualitative case study.
Survey research	A database records allegations/instances of abuse of vulnerable children reported by schools and social services.
Experimental research	Vicky appeared to ask Marion to provide her with medication to relieve her feelings of being 'stressed out'. Such medication would have been developed via scientific controlled trials.

Further reading

Standing, M (2023) *Clinical Judgement and Decision-Making in Nursing* (5th edn). London: SAGE.

In-depth application of the matrix model. A chapter is devoted to each of the ten perceptions of clinical decision-making in nursing, cross-referenced to ten conceptions of nursing, which are demonstrated using case studies. There is also a more detailed account of the 'PERSON' evaluation tool and its applications.

Ellis, P (2023) *Evidence-based Practice in Nursing* (5th edn). London: SAGE.

Clearly explains the wide range of evidence informing nursing practice and how it is applied. Chapter 7 contains another worked example of applying the PERSON evaluation tool.

Price, B (2022) *Delivering Person-centred Care in Nursing* (2nd edn). London: SAGE.

Detailed account of what person-centred care is and how to apply and refine it in practice.

Useful websites

www.nice.org.uk

National Institute for Health and Care Excellence website, where you can find a wide variety of evidence-based assessment tools and clinical guidelines.

https://www.nhs.uk/conditions/nhs-screening/

NHS website identifies the eleven national screening programmes promoting preventative healthcare, including abdominal aortic aneurysm (AAA) screening as discussed in the chapter.

https://www.local.gov.uk/our-support/our-improvement-offer/care-and-health-improvement

Local Government Association website explaining Local Authorities' remit for preventative physical and mental healthcare, social care provision, and tackling health inequalities.

Glossary

Abdominal aortic aneurysm (AAA): swelling in the aorta between the heart and the pelvis that may require surgical intervention to prevent it rupturing or to urgently repair a rupture.

Acculturate: become assimilated into a new (dominant) culture.

Anaemia: lack of haemoglobin, which lowers the oxygen-carrying capacity of the red blood cells.

Arteriogram: injection of substance that shows up on X-ray to outline arterial vessels.

Autonomy: the ability to exercise choice.

Beneficence: the ethical principle of doing good.

Body language: body movements and expressions that reveal emotions.

Cerebrovascular accident (CVA): also known as a stroke, this is an interruption to blood flow in a vessel in the brain due to either a clot or rupture.

Clinical decision-making: applies clinical judgement to select the best possible evidence-based option to control risks and address patients' needs in high-quality care for which you are accountable.

Clinical judgement: informed opinion (using intuition, reflection and critical thinking) that relates observation and assessment of patients to identifying and evaluating alternative nursing options.

Closed question: questions that illicit a short, often one-word, answer.

Cognitive continuum: judgement, ranging from intuitive hunches to critical analysis, that is tailored to the constantly changing nature of clinical demands and health problems we deal with.

Consequentialism: the ethical theory that regards the ends as justifying the means.

Cruse: bereavement support service.

Delirious: suffering from confusion caused by fever.

Deontology: this is about rule-based ethics.

Electrocardiogram (ECG): a procedure that records the electrical activity of the heart and produces a tracing of this.

Epigastric pain: pain in the upper abdominal region.

Exudate: leakage from a wound.

Fibroadenoma: a collection of fibrous and glandular cells that form a mobile lump with distinct boundaries.

Glasgow Coma Scale: a neurological scale that measures levels of consciousness.

Glucocorticoids: a group of hormones released by the adrenal cortex.

Holistic: taking into account the whole person: physical, mental, social and spiritual.

Hypoglycaemia: low blood sugar level.

Idiocultures: the knowledge systems and ways of behaving of a small group of people.

Ingest: eat or drink.

Intuition/intuitive: the ability to subconsciously use information cues to make sense of a situation.

Justice: the principle of treating people fairly.

Leading question: a question that suggests what the answer to it is.

Lifeworld: the world as experienced by an individual.

Mindfulness: focusing on and becoming acutely aware of things normally taken for granted.

Neurological: arising from the nervous system.

Neuropathy: loss of peripheral sensation, particularly in the feet, due to damaged nerve endings and reduced blood flow.

Non-maleficence: the ethical principle of not doing harm.

Objective: refers to things that can be measured in some way.

Oesophageal gastroduodenoscopy (OGD):   a procedure in which a flexible tube with a camera is passed through the oesophagus, stomach and duodenum to visualise the internal lining and structure.

Open question: a question that allows the person answering to choose what and how much they say.

'PERSON' evaluation tool: a new universal framework to question, evaluate and guide nursing and midwifery decisions/interventions in the six key areas, namely **p**atient-centred; **e**vidence-based; **r**isks assessed and managed; **s**afe and effective delivery of care; **o**utcomes benefit the patient; and **n**ursing and midwifery strengths and weaknesses.

Primary prevention: preventing illness, disease or injury from occurring in the first place through targeted measures, for example, fluoridation of water to reduce incidence of tooth decay.

Prognosis: predicted course of the disease.

Quantitative: things that can be counted/quantified.

Secondary prevention: early detection and intervention in health problems to reduce their impact and aid recovery; for example, mammography screening enables breast cancer to be identified and treated.

Stent: a corrugated metal or plastic cylindrical tube inserted into a vessel to maintain its patency.

Subjective: information and understandings that are based on personal opinion.

Sympathetic presence: employing empathy to understand a patient's needs in a person-centred way.

Symptom: a manifestation of a disease that the patient experiences but which cannot be seen or measured directly.

Tertiary prevention: Managing longer term health problems and disabilities to prevent further complications arising, for example, ongoing support to make lifestyle adjustments in diet, exercise, alcohol consumption.

Ulcerative colitis: inflammatory disease of the large bowel.

Urisheath: a device that covers the penis, directing urine into a tube which empties into a bag.

Values: the beliefs that are attached to a desirable outcome of a particular action.

References

Ackley, BJ, Ladwig, GB, Makic, MB, Martinez-Kratz, M and Zanotti, M (2022) *Nursing Diagnosis Handbook E-Book: An Evidence-Based Guide to Planning Care* (12th edn). St Louis: Elsevier.

Aggleton, P and Chalmers, H (2000) *Nursing Models and Nursing Practice* (2nd edn). Basingstoke: Palgrave.

Andrews, J and Butler, M (2014) *Trusted to Care*. Available at: http://wales.gov.uk/docs/dhss/publications/140512trustedtocareen.pdf.

Anthony, D (2010) Do risk assessment scales for pressure ulcers work? *Journal of Tissue Viability*, *19*(4): 132–6.

Aston, L, Wakefield, J and McGown, R (eds) (2010) *The Student Nurse Guide to Decision Making in Practice*. Maidenhead: Open University Press.

Barker, J (2013) *Evidence-Based Practice for Nurses* (2nd edn). London: SAGE.

Baumbusch, J, Leblanc, M-E, Shaw, M and Kjorven, M (2016) Factors influencing nurses' readiness to care for hospitalised older people. *International Journal of Older People Nursing*, *11*(2): 149–59.

Beauchamp, T and Childress, J (2013) *Principles of Biomedical Ethics* (7th edn). Oxford: Oxford University Press.

Bender, M (2017) Models versus theories as a primary carrier of nursing knowledge: A philosophical argument. *Nursing Philosophy 19*:e12198 https://doi.org/10.1111/nup.12198

Benjamin, M and Curtis, J (2010) *Ethics in Nursing* (4th edn). Oxford: Oxford University Press.

Bradley, P, Frost, F, Tharmaratnam, K and the NW Collaborative Organisation for Respiratory Research (2020) Utility of established prognostic scores in COVID-19 hospital admissions: multicentre prospective evaluation of CURB-65, NEWS2 and qSOFA. *BMJ Open Respiratory Research 7*:e000729 doi: 10.1136/bmjresp-2020-000729.

Brinkmann, S and Kvale, S (2014) *InterViews: learning the craft of qualitative research interviewing* (3rd edn). London: SAGE.

Burbach, B, Barnason, S and Thompson, SA (2015) Using 'think aloud' to capture clinical reasoning during patient simulation. *International Journal of Nurse Education and Scholarship*, *3*: 12: doi: 10.1515/ijnes-2014-0044

Caldeira, S, Timmins, F, Carvalho, EC and Vieira, M (2017) Clinical validation of the nursing diagnosis spiritual distress. *International Journal of Nursing Terminology and Knowledge*, *28*(1): 44–52.

Care Quality Commission (CQC) (2022) Out of sight – who cares? Restraint, segregation and seclusion review: Progress report March 2022. Available at: https://www.cqc.org.uk/sites/default/files/20220325_rssreview-progress-march_print.pdf

Carpenito-Moyet, LJ (2016) *Handbook of Nursing Diagnosis* (15th edn). Philadelphia, PA: Wolters Kluwer Health/Lippincott Williams Wilkins.

Carper, B (1978) Fundamental patterns of knowing in nursing. *Advances in Nursing Science, 1*(1): 13–24.

Clark, M, Semple, MJ, Ivins, N, Mahoney, K and Herding, K (2017) National audit of pressure ulcers and incontinence-associated dermatitis in hospitals across Wales: a cross-sectional study. *BMJ Open,* 7:e015616 doi: 10.1136/bmjopen-2016-015616.

Clarke, J (2013) *Spiritual Care in Everyday Nursing Practice: A New Approach.* Basingstoke: Palgrave Macmillan.

Cook, N, Shepherd, A and Boore, J (2021) *Essentials of Anatomy and Physiology for Nursing Practice* (2nd edn). London: SAGE.

Creswell, J and Poth, CN (2017) *Qualitative Inquiry and Research Design: Choosing among Five Approaches* (4th edn). Thousand Oaks, CA: SAGE.

D'Agostino, F, Pancani, L, Romero-Sánchez, JM, Lumillo-Gutierrez, I, Paloma-Castro, O, Vellone, E, et al. (2018) Nurses' beliefs about nursing diagnosis: a study with cluster analysis. *Journal of Advanced Nursing, 74*(6): 1359–70.

D'Agostino, F, Sanson, G, Cocchieri, A, Vellone, E, Welton, J, Maurici, M, et al. (2017) Prevalence of nursing diagnoses as a measure of nursing complexity in a hospital setting. *Journal of Advanced Nursing, 73*(9): 2129–42.

Department of Health (2010a) *Equity and Excellence: Liberating the NHS.* Available at: https://assets.publishing.service.gov.uk/government/uploads/system/uploads/attachment_data/file/213823/dh_117794.pdf

Department of Health and NHS Commissioning Board (DH and NHS CB) (2012) *Compassion in Practice: Nursing, Midwifery and Care Staff, Our Vision and Strategy.* Available at: www.england.nhs.uk/wp-content/uploads/2012/12/compassion-in-practice.pdf

Dewing, J (2004) Concerns relating to the application of frameworks to promote person-centredness in nursing with older people. *Journal of Clinical Nursing, 13*(3a): 39–44.

Dewing, J (2008) Personhood and dementia: revisiting Tom Kitwood's ideas. *International Journal of Older People Nursing, 3*(1): 3–13.

Dougherty, L, Lister, S and West-Oram, A (eds) (2015) *The Royal Marsden Hospital Manual of Clinical Nursing Procedures Student Edition* (9th edn). Oxford: Wiley-Blackwell.

Dyson, S (2004) Transcultural nursing care of adults. In C. Husband and B. Terry (eds), *Transcultural Health Care Practice: An Educational Resource for Nurses and Health Care Practitioners.* London: RCN.

Egan, G (2014) *The Skilled Helper: A Problem-Management and Opportunity Development Approach to Helping* (10th edn). Belmont, CA: Brooks/Cole.

Ellis, P (2019) The meaning of consequentialism. *Journal of Kidney Care 4*(5): 274–76.

Ellis, P (2020) *Understanding Ethics for Nursing Students* (3rd edn). London: SAGE.

Ellis, P (2023) *Evidence-Based Practice in Nursing* (5th edn). London: SAGE.

Equality and Human Rights Commission (EHRC) (2011) *Inquiry into Home Care of Older People.* Available at: www.equalityhumanrights.com/legal-and-policy/our-legal-work/inquiries-and-assessments/inquiry-into-home-care-of-older-people

Esterhuizen, P (2022) *Reflective Practice in Nursing* (5th edn). London: SAGE.

Field, L and Smith, B (2008) *Nursing Care: An Essential Guide.* Harlow: Pearson Education.

Francis, R (2013) *Report of the Mid Staffordshire NHS Foundation Trust Public Inquiry: Executive Summary.* Available at: www.midstaffspublicinquiry.com/sites/default/files/report/Executive%20summary.pdf

Frosh, S (2002) *After Words: The Personal in Gender, Culture and Psychotherapy.* Basingstoke: Palgrave.

Funkesson, KH, Anbäcken, EM and Ek, AC (2007) Nurses' reasoning process during care planning taking pressure ulcer prevention as an example: a think-aloud study. *International Journal of Nursing Studies, 44*(7): 1109–19.

Girard, NJ (2007) Do you know what you don't know? *AORN Journal, 86*: 177–8.

Goodhand, K and Ewen, J (2022) Assisting people with their nutritional needs, in Delves-Yates, C (ed) *Essentials of Nursing Practice* (3rd edn). London: SAGE.

Goodman, B and Clemow, R (2010) *Nursing and Collaborative Practice: A Guide to Interprofessional Learning and Working* (2nd edn). Exeter: Learning Matters.

Gordon, M (1994) *Nursing Diagnosis: Process and Application.* St Louis, MO: Mosby Yearbook.

Grant, A and Goodman, B (2018) *Communication and Interpersonal Skills in Nursing* (4th edn). London: SAGE.

Hall, C and Ritchie, D (2013) *What Is Nursing? Exploring Theory and Practice* (3rd edn). London: SAGE.

Hammond, KR (1996) *Human Judgement and Social Policy: Irreducible Uncertainty, Inevitable Error, Unavoidable Injustice.* New York: Oxford University Press.

Hawkey, B and Williams, J (2007) *The Role after Rehabilitation Nurse: RCN Guidance.* London: RCN.

Healthcare Improvement Scotland (HIS) (2021) *People-Led Care Portfolio.* Available at: https://ihub.scot/improvement-programmes/people-led-care/

Heron, J (1992) *Feeling and Personhood: Psychology in Another Key.* London: SAGE.

Hill, TE (2010) How clinicians make (or avoid) moral judgments of patients: implications of the evidence for relationships and research. *Philosophy, Ethics, and Humanities in Medicine, 5*(11) doi:10.1186/1747-5341-5-11

Hillson, D and Murray-Webster, R (2007) *Understanding and Managing Risk Attitude* (2nd edn). Farnham: Gower.

Hinchliff, S, Norman, S and Schober, J (eds) (2008) *Nursing Practice and Health Care* (5th edn). London: Hodder Arnold.

Holland, K and Jenkins, J (2019) *Applying the Roper, Logan and Tierney Model in Practice* (3rd edn). London: Churchill Livingstone.

Holmes, S (2010) Importance of nutrition in palliative care of patients with chronic disease. *Nursing Standard, 25*(1): 48–56.

Howatson-Jones, L and Ellis, P (eds) (2008) *Outpatient, Day Surgery and Ambulatory Care.* Chichester: Wiley-Blackwell.

Hubley, J and Copeman, J (2013) *Practical Health Promotion* (2nd edn). Cambridge: Polity Press.

Hutchfield, K (2010) *Information Skills for Nursing Students.* Exeter: Learning Matters.

Ikäheimo, H and Laitinen, A (2007) Dimensions of personhood. *Journal of Consciousness Studies, 14*(5–6): 6–16.

Innes, A, Macpherson, S and McCabe, L (2006) *Promoting Person-Centred Care at the Frontline.* York: Joseph Rowntree Foundation.

Kahneman, D (2011) *Thinking, Fast and Slow.* New York: Farrar, Straus and Giroux.

Kara, A, DeMeester, D, Lazo, L, Cook, E and Hendricks, S (2018) An interprofessional patient assessment involving medical and nursing students: a qualitative study. *Journal of Interprofessional Care, 32*(4): 513–16, https://doi.org/10.1080/13561820.2018.1442821

Keogh, B (2013) *Review into the Quality of Care and Treatment Provided by 14 Hospital Trusts in England: Overview Report.* Available at: www.nhs.uk/NHSEngland/bruce-keogh-review/Documents/outcomes/keogh-review-final-report.pdf

Kipling, R (ND) *The Elephant's Child.* Available at: www.kiplingsociety.co.uk/rg_elephantschild1.htm

Kitwood, T (1997) *Dementia Reconsidered: The Person Comes First.* Milton Keynes: Open University Press.

Lloyd, M (2010) *A Practical Guide to Care Planning in Health and Social Care.* Maidenhead: Open University Press.

Lynch, L, Hancox, K, Happell, B and Parker, J (2008) *Clinical Supervision for Nurses.* Chichester: Wiley-Blackwell.

Mahoney, F and Barthel, D (1965) Functional evaluation: The Barthel Index. *Maryland State Medical Journal, 14:* 56–61.

Manley, K (2000) Organisational culture and consultant nurse outcomes: part 1 – organisational culture. *Nursing Standard, 14*(36): 34–8.

Manley, K and McCormack, B (2003) Practice development: purpose, methodology, facilitation and evaluation. *Nursing in Critical Care, 8*(1): 22–9.

Manley, K, Sanders, K, Cardiff, S and Webster, J (2011) Effective workplace culture: the attributes, enabling factors and consequences of a new concept. *International Practice Development Journal, 1*(2): Article 1.

McAllister, M (ed) (2007) *Solution-Focused Nursing: Rethinking Practice.* Basingstoke: Palgrave.

McCabe, C and Timmins, F (2013) *Communication Skills for Nursing Practice* (2nd edn). Basingstoke: Palgrave Macmillan.

McCaffery, M (1968) *Nursing Practice Theories Related to Cognition, Bodily Pain, and Man–Environment Interactions.* Los Angeles, CA: University of California at Los Angeles Students' Store.

McCarthy, MP and Jones, JS (2019) The Medicalization of Nursing: The Loss of a Discipline's Unique Identity. *International Journal for Human Caring, 23*(1): 101–8.

McCormack, B (2004) Person-centredness in gerontological nursing: an overview of the literature. *Journal of Clinical Nursing, 13*(3a): 31–8.

McCormack, B and McCance, T (2016) *Person-Centred Practice in Nursing and Health Care: Theory and Practice* (2nd edn). Oxford: Wiley-Blackwell.

McCormack, B, McCance, T and Maben, J (2013) Outcome evaluation in the development of person-centred practice, in McCormack, B, Manley, K and Titchen, A (eds), *Practice Development in Nursing and Healthcare* (2nd edn). Chichester: Wiley-Blackwell, pp 190–211.

Mental Capacity Act 2005. London: The Stationery Office.

Mental Health Act 2007. London: The Stationery Office.

Morris, RC (2012) The relative influence of values and identities on academic dishonesty: a quantitative analysis. *Current Research in Social Psychology, 20*(1): 1–20.

Moule, P and Goodman, M (2009) *Nursing Research: An Introduction.* London: SAGE.

National Institute for Health and Care Excellence (NICE) (2007) *Acutely Ill Patients in Hospital.* London: NICE.

National Institute for Health and Care Excellence (NICE) (2017) *Nutrition Support for Adults: Oral Nutrition Support, Enteral Tube Feeding, and Parenteral Nutrition.* London: NICE.

National Institute for Health and Care Excellence (NICE) (2020) *Abdominal aortic aneurysm: diagnosis and management [NG 156].* London: NICE.

National Institute for Health and Care Excellence (NICE) (2022) *Type 2 diabetes in adults: management: NICE guideline [NG28].* Available at: https://www.nice.org.uk/guidance/ng28

NHS (2019) *The NHS Long Term Care Plan – A Summary.* Available at: www.longtermplan.nhs.uk/wp-content/uploads/2019/01/the-nhs-long-term-plan-summary.pdf

NHS (2021) *Overview: Abdominal aortic aneurysm screening.* Available at: https://www.nhs.uk/conditions/abdominal-aortic-aneurysm-screening/

NHS Digital (2022) *Data on Written Complaints in the NHS 2021–22.* Available at: https://digital.nhs.uk/data-and-information/publications/statistical/data-on-written-complaints-in-the-nhs/2020-21

NHS England (ND) *Involving people in their own care.* Available at: https://www.england.nhs.uk/ourwork/patient-participation/

Nightingale, F (1860) *Notes on Nursing: What It Is and What It Is Not.* New York: Appleton.

Nolan, D and Ellis, P (2008) Communication and advocacy, in Howatson-Jones, L and Ellis, P (eds) *Outpatient, Day Surgery and Ambulatory Care.* Chichester: Wiley-Blackwell, pp 8–24.

Norberg Boysen, G, Nyström, M, Christensson, L, Herlitz, J and Wireklint Sundström, B (2017) Trust in the early chain of healthcare: lifeworld hermeneutics from the patient's perspective. *International Journal of Qualitative Studies on Health and Well-being, 12*(1): https://doi.org/10.1080/17482631.2017.1356674

Northern Ireland Public Services Ombudsman (NIPSO) (2021) *Northern Ireland Public Service Ombudsman: Ombudsman's Report 2020/2021.* Available at: https://nipso.org.uk/site/wp-content/uploads/2021/11/Ombudsmans-Report-2020-21.pdf

Nursing and Midwifery Council (NMC) (2018a) *Future Nurse: Standards of Proficiency for Registered Nurses.* London: NMC.

Nursing and Midwifery Council (NMC) (2018b) *The Code: Professional Standards of Practice and Behaviour for Nurses, Midwives and Nursing Associates.* London: NMC.

Ogden, K, Barr, J and Greenfield, D (2017) Determining requirements for patient-centred care: a participatory concept mapping study. *BMC Health Service Research, 17*: 780 https://doi.org/10.1186/s12913-017-2741-y

Orem, D (2001) *Nursing: Concepts of Practice* (6th edn). London: Mosby.

Park, C (2007) *A Dictionary of Environment and Conservation* (3rd edn). Oxford: Oxford University Press.

Peate, I (2019) *Learning to Care: The Nurse Associate.* London: Elsevier.

Price, B (2022) *Delivering Person-Centred Care in Nursing* (2nd edn). London: SAGE.

Pritchard, MJ (2011) Using the Hospital Anxiety and Depression Scale in surgical patients. *Nursing Standard, 25*(34): 35–41.

Public Health England (PHE) (2017) *NHS Abdominal Aortic Aneurysm (AAA) Screening Programme.* London: PHE.

Rahman, S and Myers, R (2019) *Courage in Healthcare: A Necessary Virtue or a Warning Sign?* London: SAGE.

Ringdal, M, Chaboyer, W, Ulin, K, Bucknall, T and Oxelmark, L (2017) Patient preferences for participation in patient care and safety activities in hospitals. *BMC Nursing, 16*: 69 https://doi.org/10.1186/s12912-017-0266-7

Rogers, C (1995) *A Way of Being.* Boston, MA: Houghton Mifflin.

Roper, N, Logan, W and Tierney, A (2000) *The Roper–Logan–Tierney Model of Nursing: Based on Activities of Living.* Edinburgh: Churchill Livingstone.

Rosen, M (2021) *Many Different Kinds of Love: A Story of Life, Death and the NHS.* London: Ebury Press.

Royal College of Nursing (RCN) (2003) *Defining Nursing.* London: RCN.

Royal College of Physicians (RCP) (2012) *National Early Warning Score (NEWS): Standardising the Assessment of Acute-Illness Severity in the NHS.* Available at: www.rcplondon.ac.uk/national-early-warning-score

Sakamoto, ML (2018) Nursing knowledge: A middle ground exploration. *Nursing Philosophy, 19*(3):e12209 https://doi.org/10.1111/nup.12209

Schwartz, SH (1992) Universals in the content and structure of values: theoretical advances and empirical tests in 20 countries, in Zanna, MP (ed) *Advances in Experimental Social Psychology.* London: Academic Press.

Scottish Public Services Ombudsman (SPSO) (2022) *Investigation Reports.* Available at: www.spso.org.uk/investigation-reports

Shah, RA, Soo, Z, Thornhill, J, Martin, J and Montagu, A (2022) Improving inpatient assessment of nutritional status using the Malnutrition Universal Screening Tool (MUST). *Proceedings of the Nutrition Society, 81*(OCE3): E79. Available at: https://doi.org/10.1017/S0029665122001045

Social Care Institute for Excellence (ND) *Person-centred care.* Available at: https://www.scie.org.uk/prevention/choice/person-centred-care

Social Care Institute for Excellence (2020) *Types and indicators of abuse 2020.* Available at: https://www.scie.org.uk/safeguarding/adults/introduction/types-and-indicators-of-abuse

Sorenson, C, Bolick, B, Wright, K and Hamilton, R (2016) Understanding compassion fatigue in healthcare providers: a review of current literature. *Journal of Nursing Scholarship, 48*(5): 456–65.

Standing, M (2010) *Clinical Judgement and Decision Making.* Maidenhead: Open University Press.

Standing, M (2023) *Clinical Judgement and Decision Making in Nursing* (5th edn). London: SAGE.

Stephenson, J (2014) *NHS England to Rollout '6Cs' Nursing Values to All Health Service Staff.* Available at: www.nursingtimes.net/nursing-practice/specialisms/management/exclusive-6cs-nursing-values-to-be-rolled-out-to-all-nhs-staff/5070102.article.

Stets, JE and Carter, MJ (2011) The moral self: applying identity theory. *Social Psychology Quarterly, 74*(2): 192–215.

Stiles, KA (2011) Advancing nursing knowledge through complex holism. *ANS Adv Nurs Sci 34*(1):39–50. Available at: https://doi.org/10.1097/ANS.0b013e31820943b9

Suhonen, R, Stolt, M, Habermann, M, Hjaltadottir, I, Vryonides, S, Tonnessen, S, Halvorsen, K, Harvey, C, Toffoli, L and Scott, PA (2018) Ethical elements in priority setting in nursing care: A scoping review. *International Journal of Nursing Studies, 88*: 25–42. Available at: https://doi.org/10.1016/j.ijnurstu.2018.08.006

Sully, P and Dallas, J (2010) *Essential Communication Skills for Nursing and Midwifery* (2nd edn). Edinburgh: Elsevier Mosby.

Vincent, JL, Einav, S, Pearse, R, Jaber, S, Kranke, P, Overdyk, FJ, Whitaker, DK, Gordo, F, Dahan, A and Hoeft, A (2018) Improving detection of patient deterioration in the general hospital ward environment. *European Journal of Anaesthesiology, 35*(5):325–33 https://doi.org/10.1097/EJA.0000000000000798

Waterlow, J (2008) *The Waterlow Score.* Available at: www.judy-waterlow.co.uk

Weir-Hughes, D (2007) Reviewing nursing diagnoses. *Nursing Management, 14*(5): 32–5.

Welton, JM and Halloran, EJ (2005) Nursing diagnoses, diagnosis-related group, and hospital outcomes. *Journal of Nursing Administration, 35*(12): 541–9.

West, L, Alheit, P, Anderson, AS and Merrill, B (eds) (2007) *Using Biographical and Life History Approaches in the Study of Adult and Lifelong Learning: European Perspectives.* Frankfurt am Main: Peter Lang.

Wilkinson, JM (2016) *Nursing Diagnosis Handbook* (11th edn). Harlow: Pearson Education.

Wilson, B, Woollands, A and Barrett, D (2018) *Care Planning: A Guide for Nurses* (3rd edn). Harlow: Pearson Education.

Worden, A and Challis, D (2008) Care planning systems in care homes for older people. *Quality in Ageing, 8*: 28–38.

World Health Organization (WHO) (2018) Low quality healthcare is increasing the burden of illness and health costs globally. Available at: https://www.who.int/news/item/05-07-2018-low-quality-healthcare-is-increasing-the-burden-of-illness-and-health-costs-globally

Index

Locators in **bold** refer to tables

Ingram Content Group UK Ltd.
Milton Keynes UK
UKHW051915190423
420450UK00001B/9